PRAISE FOR
TO EXIST AS I AM

'Grace Spence Green is an essential voice in the conversation on anti-ableism and true representation'
Shani Dhanda

'Exquisitely written and compelling, this book tells the story of a remarkable doctor. By the end it will have upended the preconceptions many of us hold as to what it is to lead a rich, fulfilled life'
Caroline Elton

'A story of injury, loss and acceptance that asks us to consider what it truly means to recover. Grace Spence Green shows us how much we can gain when we stop trying to overcome disability and start embracing it as part of what makes us human. Her story is inspiring in the best possible ways: as an activist call to arms and a testament to the joy that comes through finding your community'
David Turner

'Astonishing, important and truly radical. In picking apart so many of the tired binaries we use to think about love, care, trauma and healing, it is as if – at last – someone had switched the lights on. Lucid and hopeful but also fierce in its challenge to a world that so often gets disability all wrong, this book is completely transformative'
Polly Morland

To Exist As I Am

wellcome collection

WELLCOME COLLECTION is a free museum and library near Euston station in London. We believe everyone's experience of health matters. Through our collections, exhibitions and events, in books and online, we explore the past, present and future of health.

We care for many thousands of items relating to health, medicine and human experience, including rare books, artworks, films and videos, personal archives, and objects. We're part of Wellcome, a charitable foundation supporting science to help build a healthier future for everyone.

To Exist As I Am

*A Doctor's Notes on Recovery
and Radical Acceptance*

Grace Spence Green

P

PROFILE BOOKS

wellcome
collection

First published in Great Britain in 2025 by
Profile Books Ltd
29 Cloth Fair
London
ECIA 7JQ
www.profilebooks.com

Published in association with Wellcome Collection

183 Euston Road
London NW1 2BE
www.wellcomecollection.org

Typeset in Sabon by CC Book Production

1 3 5 7 9 10 8 6 4 2

Printed and bound in Great Britain by
CPI Group (UK) Ltd, Croydon, CR0 4YY

A CIP catalogue record for this book is available from the British Library.

We make every effort to make sure our products are safe for the purpose
for which they are intended. For more information check our website or contact
Authorised Rep Compliance Ltd., Ground Floor, 71 Lower Baggot Street,
Dublin, D02 P593, Ireland, www.arccompliance.com

ISBN 978 1 80081 4486
eISBN 978 1 80081 4493

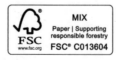

For Nathan and my parents

I exist as I am, that is enough,
If no other in the world be aware I sit content,
And if each and all be aware I sit content.

One world is aware and by far the largest to me,
    and that is myself,
And whether I come to my own today or in ten
    thousand or ten million years,
I can cheerfully take it now, or with equal cheerfulness
    I can wait.

Walt Whitman, 'Song of Myself'

Prologue

'You make the past known in order to know yourself as changed'

– Melissa Febos

'Is that what you've got then?'

She is looking at me closely, pointing to a red circular badge I have attached to my lanyard that reads *'Ask me about 22Q!'*

22Q is a rare genetic syndrome (which I do not have), causing a range of health conditions, affecting very cute children. I have just finished a research project on it at the children's hospital next door.

I curse myself for wearing the badge and try to think of any way to avoid the line of questioning I know is coming. I brace myself.

We are sitting in a rheumatology clinic, and I find myself in the situation every medical student dreads – the consultant has left the room 'for just a minute', leaving me and the patient to make small talk.

I glance anxiously at the door, wishing they would come back. *I don't want to be here. I don't even like bones!* I think.

'No!' I smile brightly in response to her question.

'What have you got then?'

'A spinal cord injury,' I say, and I don't know why I say it. I'm hoping she won't ask the next question that I know is coming, that I am *naive* to think won't be next. But we are already there.

'What happened to you?'

It's a funny thing when you realise how blurred the line between doctor and patient can be. But I am learning that this is how I interact with the world now, which is suddenly unsure where to place me. Sometimes because of anxiety or awkwardness. Sometimes I sense real fear.

We have reversed roles. I was silly to think I would be the only one asking the questions today (or at least listening to her answers, while my consultant takes charge). My own intimate medical past is also up for grabs, apparently.

Before I can begin to formulate a response, she's brought up suggestions.

'Was it a car crash? Oh, it was a car crash, wasn't it? What happened then? Did you fall? I hope you weren't being silly. What happened to you?'

This is a daily occurrence now, while I'm desperately trying to be taken seriously on wards and in clinics, in hospital corridors.

What *happened* to you? What's *wrong* with you? Is it *permanent*?

Why are you in a wheelchair?

How do I begin? I sigh at having to start here, always. It's a story I have told thousands of times, by now. So, let's get it over with.

Although it wasn't a car crash, I was a part of a collision.

It was mid-afternoon, October 2018, at Westfield shopping centre in London. I was in my fourth year of medical school at the time. As is the standard practice at large London medical schools, we had been shipped off to various places outside the city for four months 'on peripheral'. I was living in Maidstone as part of my Women's Health placement, flitting between Maidstone and Tunbridge Wells hospitals. I had been allocated there with three of my closest friends. It was my first time seeing a birth. I was feeling more confident, now in my second year of clinical placements, even if the extent of my involvement was holding a retractor to pull the skin away during an operation, cutting excess thread from sewn surgical stitches, writing a freshly born baby's name for the first time on a tiny patient wristband.

We only had a few more weeks left before we would move back to London. I had a coaching shift in the city at the climbing centre I worked at for extra money, so my friend drove me in, dropping me off at a shopping centre so I could catch the tube up to Manor House.

Events here become a collection of moments, and sometimes I don't trust myself on their accuracy. How can you be sure if you remember something, or if you're imagining a memory because you've been told it happened so many times with so many different variations? Because you've seen it written down on official documents, drawn up by important people, and so have taken it as fact?

My friend and I hugged goodbye at the escalators,

planning to meet up later. I was walking down the atrium towards the train station when the collision occurred.

I awoke to find myself lying on the floor of the shopping centre.

The strangest part was waking up for the second time that day, not realising I had been unconscious. Someone was holding my head still, tightly. Faces drifted in and out of my view. The adrenaline jolted me wide awake. Thoughts frantically flickered through my mind in those first minutes. I told the faces that they need to call my partner, to call my parents. I told them my phone is in my bag.

I began to sense that there was another person lying near me. Were they a part of this? They were telling this figure he fell from the third floor. I found out later that he jumped.

I realised at that point that I could not feel my legs. No, this phrasing isn't entirely accurate; it's not that I couldn't feel them, it's that my legs didn't feel anything back. As if they had ceased to exist.

The collision had broken my spine, causing bone to press into my spinal cord, paralysing me from the chest down. Multiple breaks, in fact, but I would only find this out much later.

How surreal it is to read your own MRI report years on, finding out injuries you didn't even realise you had. Like a plug yanked from its socket, I had been disconnected from the lower half of my body in an instant.

I remember crying, maybe screaming.

And in that moment the life that I had mapped out so well, so clearly, no longer appeared in front of me. It fell away to reveal a nothingness. The tracks had changed, I was on a new course.

Everything was different now.

While the sequence of events themselves may be simple – and may be all that strangers want to hear – what has come to mean so much more to me, what I really want people to understand, is what came after. I have spent the years since being discharged trying to find a new place in the world, a new community, a new identity.

I like to think taking a history from a patient is a guided storytelling, stories we can take and compile into clues to help treat someone. Lots of what I do at work involves listening to stories every day, and from there forming a plan to treat or support. Now I have a story that others ask *me* about, without the justification of any real therapeutic purpose or action.

I sometimes want to respond to the enquiries of strangers with: why do you want to know? Or more importantly, why do you think it's acceptable to ask this question so casually, so flippantly, to me or any other visibly disabled person? How would you feel if I asked you to recount the most traumatic events of your life, every time you meet someone new?

Do I scare you? I want to ask. Does my appearance frighten you?

These questions are so often framed as harmless curiosity, but for some it seems to be the only way to interact with me, the only thing I can talk about now, the only thing people are interested in. As if I am in a permanent state of acute illness. I want people to understand what it's like to be plagued almost daily by such questions up front, before all else; to know what it feels like to have your life decided, defined by a singular day, a day you remember so little of. In taxis, in the pub, in lifts.

My medical training had coached me to look for clues and signs in other people's bodies to trace the root of disease, but suddenly it's my own body that's medicalised at every turn.

In this way, I am reminded regularly that to others there must be something inherently *wrong* with the way that I am. It makes me feel like an alien; people need to know where I have come from. My backstory must be revealed, because the mystery is disconcerting.

My body has somehow become something to explain right away, to ease other people's discomfort. A wheelchair, it turns out, is the elephant of all elephants in the room. I cannot simply *exist*.

How many gasps and wide-eyed faces can I take in? How many times can I hear how tragic, how awful, how dreadful, how terrible, how devastating my circumstances are? How many times can I hear these words before I start to believe them?

For a long time, I felt defined by a sensational headline. An anecdote for strangers to take back home and tell others: my life, summed up in a handful of sentences.

I am tired, too, of answering questions about the man who jumped, not just because I barely know the answers – I haven't even seen him since. It can feel like my life is being reduced to this single moment, forever tied to a stranger. It colours everything, a muddy lens over my screen. I cannot escape it. I am so tired of talking about that day.

I have had enough of watching my identity being boiled down to a story that someone else has chosen for me.

I no longer want to feel as though I am suffocating, existing as a disabled person in a society that has such a strict, preformed idea of what that means. I so badly want to be received respectfully, openly, without judgement, without a voyeurism that frequently tips over into something morbid.

My own time as an inpatient, and then being out in the world as a visibly disabled person, has radicalised me. I soon realised how I and other disabled people are systematically excluded, both passively and actively. That I have specific spaces I am allowed to enter, and specific narratives I am allowed to follow – tropes to fall in with. And this, coupled with the constant intrusive questions, the denial of privacy and dignity, the automatic pathologising of my body now I am seated, all conveyed to me the message that I now exist for others.

Early on, I began to look critically at the social infrastructure I was brought up in, one that was only reinforced by years of medical study, that taught me so much about what can go 'wrong' and what needs to be 'fixed'.

I began to understand that everything I had been taught about disabled people, about what it means to be well or sick, for the past twenty-two years needed to be undone, unpicked. In fact, it very quickly began to unravel before my eyes. These changes were scary, but also felt powerful and necessary.

In those early days, I read and scavenged and learned, like I was revising for the most important exam of my life. I had to start from scratch on myself. The more I learned, the more surprised I was that so few in the mainstream media were talking about disability, anti-ableism, while ashamed that even as a doctor it had taken my own injury to shift my perspective.

Words like recovery, independence and fairness took on new meanings for me.

The world shrank and then expanded, as if a mirror had been turned around to reveal a window. I began to redraw the lines between well and unwell, to reconsider definitions of health and the extent to which my body is impaired, and the ways in which society impairs me. I have been forging an entirely new relationship with my body, as I see many of my patients do, after major operations, drastic physical changes, illness, or simply the passage of time. I have seen how, to a greater or lesser degree, we're all grappling with transformation, change, grief. I've seen what healing looks like, the different shapes it takes, and where it takes us.

In those early days after my injury my anger also fuelled hope. I was getting angry enough to realise that I deserved to be treated better, angry enough to push back.

But through all this change, I was also experiencing so much joy, such deep connection with others, so much strength. I was coming to an acceptance of myself, all while navigating grief and my own internalised ableism. I understood that so much of what allowed me to progress and to recover was thanks to my community, and the privileges of being white, middle class and financially secure. That so many others in my circumstances and across the disabled community lacked the essential resources to do this.

I'm desperate to find better ways to have conversations about disability. Conversations that do not feel so one-dimensional, so transactional. That allow space for fragility, vulnerability, strength, complexity and the breadth of human experience.

If I had the time, if I had the space, if I had the energy, maybe these encounters with strangers could go differently. I began to realise that in the fleeting moments of these interactions, when I was given five minutes to explain the intricacies of my feelings, I was doing myself a disservice. I could not begin to describe the fractures and shifts in my understanding, in my perspective, which had taken months and years to process. How could I convey such complex, confounding feelings when they sometimes felt too big to hold in my head?

Instead, I wrote. I've been chronicling my life ever since my injury: examining it, squirrelling details away in phone notes, scribbles on scrap paper, long outpourings in notebooks, quick lines in between ward rounds, emails to myself. So that one day I could hand it to someone like this stranger in clinic, press it into their hands and say look, read this please. It's all in here.

This book is a response to the thousands of interactions I have had where I didn't have the words, yet.

I loved to write and draw as a child; sketching strangers

9

on the tube to school every morning, writing bad poetry and overblown love letters to my teenage boyfriend. The demands of medical school meant I had not written for years, but five days into my hospital stay, as soon as I could type again, I began a diary. I opened my laptop, my wrists still bruised purple and green by cannulas, metal staples still holding me together. It was the only thing that kept me anchored to a new, disconcerting reality, trying to grapple with huge concepts that I'd had the privilege of never considering before.

Stories of disabling injuries that I read were sometimes helpful to me in those early days, but too often felt individual, always focused on a narrative of personal overcoming, rather than looking critically at the context that made people feel that disability was something that needed to be overcome in the first place. Something shameful, something wrong.

I want my story to be seen in the context of a greater struggle. Of generations of disabled people. In the community where I have found a place. I want it to be bigger than myself and part of a movement of collective action and solidarity that we can all play a part in.

I want you to understand the nuances of my story, and that there is nuance to disability. Disability is too often oversimplified, sensationalised or glorified, leaving no room for its dynamic nature and the rich variety of experience. I want to frame this book in hope, too, writing from a place of compassion and empathy rather than criticism. I'm writing as someone who has not always done the right thing either, or always known what might be the right thing to do – or the right words to say. I want us all to do better.

At first, those early hospital diaries I wrote were so raw, angry, confused, muddled. It is painful to go back there. It is hard to remember that time when nothing felt solid, but I think it is important to chart the journey across the chasm, from where I was to where I am now. To trace my journey back to the other side of the bed.

My body may have changed that October day, but I didn't. I was remoulded, grown over time. New ideas sprouting inside me like buds, incubating and blossoming.

To me, it's never really been about what happened that day. It's everything that happened afterwards.

PART 1:
Aftermath

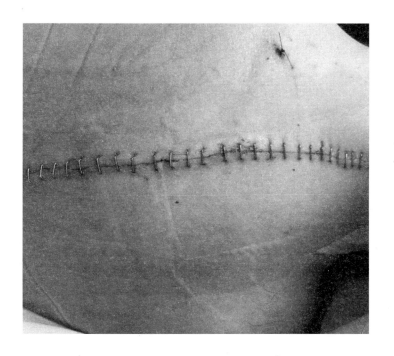

Admission

17 October 2018

Trauma call, brought in by London Ambulance Service

Mechanism of injury:

While in a shopping centre, man jumped from THIRD? 1st floor balcony – on to the patient herself. Patient does not have any recollection of the event. Woke up to find people surrounding her

Background:

4th Year medical student at Kings College Diamond-Blackfan anaemia previously requiring blood transfusion

On arrival to ED resuscitations:

GCS 15 but not moving her legs and reporting complete loss of sensation from her mid chest down to feet. Primary survey: no obvious external injuries identified

Examination of her limbs:

Upper limbs: normal tone, reflex, sensation to light touch and coordination

Lower limbs: reduced tone, power (0/5), reflexes (unable to elicit), no sensation to light touch (from T5 level downwards. No proprioception either)

ED belongings:

No valuables with patient. All clothes cut off

This is how it began. At that moment, I couldn't begin to imagine the three months that stretched ahead of me. An intensity of human experience that I had not yet known was possible.

I lay on a cold, hard hospital bed in the Royal London A&E on the evening of the 17th of October 2018. My boyfriend, Nathan, had rushed to the hospital as soon as he got the call. He could see the man who jumped and landed on me lying in the bay next to mine. He couldn't see his face; only his legs, which were moving. He was crossing one over another.

Mine were not moving, although I don't notice that then. I was more concerned that my friend had to get back home from here late at night. *Call her an Uber* I whispered loudly to my mum.

I was talking very fast. It was simultaneously too bright and too dark in there. It had the aspect of a dream.

Tipsy on morphine, in that moment, I was not aware what had happened to me, what was happening to me, and what would happen to me tomorrow. I had lost all control. I had been split from a body which no longer felt like mine; others seemed to know much more about me than I did in that moment.

I couldn't tell you today who was in that room with me, how many friends visited and saw me in that state. It's something I don't like to dwell on, I would rather not know the extent of my oblivion that night.

*

When I opened my eyes again, it was the morning after my spinal cord injury.

An anaesthetist with long hair was sitting next to me. He was young and looked like someone I would be friends with, in another life. I think I must have been crying, because he said to me, 'I know, this is just shit, isn't it?'

God, I loved him for that.

It was the best thing someone could have said to me in that moment. With those few words he saw me as a whole person and appreciated the situation I now found myself in. Preparing for titanium to be bolted into my spine to hold my shattered vertebrae in place.

He had a clipboard and went through a list of questions with me, preparing to put me under general anaesthetic.

'You don't smoke, do you?' he asked casually. I looked at him wide-eyed and whispered, 'Sometimes', thinking of the one cigarette I'd tried at a party recently, terrified for some reason that this would affect everything.

He smiled and laughed. 'That's okay, we've all done that.'

Perhaps he was so important to me because he was the first doctor I remember after my injury. The first face I saw. I trusted him. My memory of him has become blurry over the years, shapes and colours with a kind voice. But his words have stayed with me.

These days, I sometimes ask myself: will people remember me like I remember him?

I had spent long enough sitting with anaesthetists as a medical student to understand how important their job is. They may get less glory than surgeons, but when things go south in the operating theatre, they are the ones in control. For the next eight hours, it would be up to him to keep me alive.

Writing this now, I run my finger over the pale dot on my wrist that sits above my radial artery, knowing there was once a wire threaded into that artery, as I lay limp.

I was called into surgery earlier than expected, and so my parents and Nathan didn't arrive in time to see me before I was moved. A nurse asked if I had anything that I want to say to them that she could pass on, as I was wheeled down the corridor to the operating theatre.

I asked her to tell them that I loved them very much. I'm sure I could have been more articulate with these last words, but it was – and remains – the truest thing I could say. In all the uncertainty of that moment, it was the one thing I knew for sure.

Much later, I learned that the surgeons had to stop mid-surgery to ask my parents, who were anxiously waiting for news, if they consented to them cutting up to the base of my skull, to check that the fractured bone at the top of my neck didn't also need to be bolted into place. Sometimes, late at night, I imagine myself, face down, layers of skin and fat and muscle splayed out to reveal my bones, waiting for the operation to restart.

When I finally came out of theatre, Nathan and my parents couldn't find me. After frantically searching up and down the hospital wards, they finally reached me, soaked in the orange iodine used to disinfect me during the operation, confused and crying.

From there, I spent the first week in the high-dependency unit, a strange, strange place. A warm, fuzzy, opioid dream. I was on patient-controlled analgesia, a button attached to a drip that meant I could click to receive a dose of morphine whenever I needed it. It was like being smothered in a warm blanket. I was barely conscious, floating on a cloud. I was so delirious I woke up one night convinced I was stranded on the side of a mountain, and I kept mistaking the nurse on shift for a friend I was living with in Maidstone.

I had no idea at the time how ill I was. There were three other patients in my bay. I couldn't see them, but I remember hearing gurgling noises at night. I was lying next to people who were dying. People came in and out of the bay, my blood pressure would drop without warning, my heart rate shooting up to compensate, and I would overheat easily. I had no control of my internal or external environment.

I was an entity; a body of inputs and outputs whose only goal was to keep producing and receiving them. An object with objectives, reduced to producing quantitative data. Every breath, every heartbeat, every bowel movement, urine output: my life and future life was now projected as various scores rated on charts.

A steady stream of doctors, nurses, psychologists, physiotherapists and policemen coming to peer over at me.

Where am I? Hell? I thought, waiting to be cleaned by a nurse in that hot, orange-lit room, swaddled in blankets, guttural noises coming from the bed next to me. *Everyone is dying around me, and I am alone.*

I returned to that very unit to visit a friend some five years after my injury and was surprised to notice how much larger the room was than I remembered, how neutral. No longer so hot and close and dark.

After four days in that orange light, once stable, I was stepped down from the high-dependency unit to a ward on the eleventh floor, mostly housing patients with strokes and brain injuries. Off the IV morphine, I became more trusting of my body; my existence no longer felt so precarious. The clouds began to clear, and I began to write every day.

My body was not my own in those next two weeks on the ward, as I was passed over from one healthcare professional to the other, to be touched and prodded and rolled and washed and carried. I needed to be turned on the clock every few hours. To be cleaned when dirty.

I was struggling to grasp the reality of what had happened, and what it all meant – what it would mean.

I remember clearly the first time I saw my scar. A cheerful junior doctor rolled me over and took a picture on my phone before he took the staples out. I looked at the screen, but I couldn't understand what I was seeing. Twenty-six metal staples from the top of my neck down to the middle of my back in a straight line, and a little stitch on the side where I'm assuming a drain was put in during the surgery. It was the neatest surgical line I'd ever seen. Was it real? Was that really my back? I didn't feel it, I still can't feel it now. It looked too straight, like it had been drawn on.

I had a bloodless injury, one that was clearly very

serious, but when I looked down at myself I didn't see anything wrong. I had woken up in a new body that looked the same as my old one.

The only thing that appeared new to me, the first thing I noticed, was a little mole above my belly button. That hadn't been there before, had it? How did that get there? I was disturbed by it.

The distance between the catastrophe I was told had occurred, and what I could see, was too vast. How was my brain supposed to bridge this gap? The surreal nature of the event, the lack of blood and bruising was all fuel for my denial.

How could I have gone through something so huge, and yet appear exactly the same? When I looked down at myself all I could see was this new mole on my stomach, and the purple bruise on my wrist from an arterial line, which faded after a few days. The only blood I saw from the injury itself was a bruise under my big toenail. I didn't know how that could have happened. Did he hit my toe on his way down? Did I fall on to it? I won't ever know the true pattern of our collision.

Staples had been run down my back like a zipper, as if I could still be undone, as if it could all still be undone. Now they had been removed, and the injury remained. The permanency had not registered in my head yet. Had not landed at its final destination.

I have a vague image of lying in the post-operative room, while waiting to go up to a ward following my operation, and asking the normally overly chatty nurse specialist if this meant I wasn't going to walk again. It was the first time I acknowledged my future. Perhaps part of me believed the operation was to 'fix' me, to make me go back to before. She was nervous and stumbled over her words. I had never seen a healthcare professional at a loss of what to say. By not saying anything, she had said it all.

On day three or four in the HDU, my charming and confident orthopaedic surgeon, Mr Bull, came to speak to my parents and me. He was the one who had drilled my spine back together. He had learned his techniques from a career as a military doctor in Afghanistan. We all developed a saviour complex around him.

He was explaining my diagnosis; *a T4/T5 spinal cord injury.* Paralysis *just below my breastbone.* I remember daring to put my right hand under the bedsheet while he was talking to touch my thigh, and shuddering. It was unreal. Feeling my leg and not feeling my hand back.

My legs had been lost in an abyss of crushed nerves; confused pathways and melded nerves creating a feeling that I was constantly vibrating. They now stretched on for miles, an infinite void of static between my chest and my feet, which I was only beginning to make the fuzzy outline of.

I remembered the first time I observed a lumbar puncture as a student, and how the junior doctor had explained to the patient that the spinal cord is made up of spindles floating in fluid. She described a lumbar puncture as like putting a wire through cooked spaghetti in water. I winced. My poor spaghetti never stood a chance.

*

I would spend many nights in that hospital bed, listening for hours to nurses talking to me about God, praying for me, telling me that I only had to believe to recover. I barely understood what I had lost.

I think back to a moment around that time when I was crying, surrounded by my family and only able to state the obvious: 'This is all very sad, isn't it?' I don't think I had any understanding *what* was sad yet. It was incomprehensible.

Sudden flashes of realisation would come over me, followed by a heavy calm, as though it was too much for my brain to handle all at once. I was shielded, small realities seeping in through the cracks.

As my brain whirred on, my body had gone into hibernation, or 'spinal shock' as it's known medically. This included the most unpleasantly termed 'flaccid paralysis', which meant my legs were not only immobile, but lacked any tone at all, and reacted to nothing. The loose limbs of a puppet. My period also stopped, and my blood pressure was consistently – sometimes dangerously – low. I like to think my body was focusing all its efforts on the mass of blood cells, immune cells, damaged bone and tissue congregating, vibrating at the place of impact in my back. The burning orb in the middle of my spine.

Friends and family could visit me freely now that I had moved to a standard ward and was not so acutely unwell. I felt a huge pressure once these visits started up, to tell them it was going to be okay, that I was fine – anything to placate their wide-eyed, tearful faces. To make them feel better about the awful situation I was in. I was split in two – smiling faces and superficial conversation in the daytime, and then the night would start: bleary eyes, lights on, nurses' chit-chat, roll me over, repeat. Incontinence. Crying in the dark. Hearing the patient with dementia opposite scream down the corridor that they were all trying to kill her, or the gangster whose head had been caved in with a baseball bat on his nightly shuffle. He would peer into my window every night. I was frightened of him until one day he gave me a small thumbs up and all fear dissipated instantly.

Soon I was allowed to be hoisted on to the chair next to my hospital bed. I was excited to be able to sit up for half an hour at a time, having spent so long horizontal.

Two healthcare workers I hadn't met before came into my room, dragging along with them a large, ungainly machine on wheels that had two large metal perpendicular arms. Hanging from them was a fabric sling, meant to hold me and lift me out of bed. I watched as they tried to work the machine, fiddling with buttons and wires. They moved on to working out which of my limbs were to go into the different loops of the sling. It was clear they were lost at this stage too and I felt no confidence in them.

Finally, they decided they had it figured out. Using the remote they turned on the machine and, like a claw grabber at a funfair taking its winnings, it slowly lifted me up. As I swung in the air, I felt myself slipping out, the slings that were supposed to be around my hips now making their way down my thighs. The harness folded me in half, my chin resting on my knees as I hung in the air.

After what felt like an eternity suspended up there, they lowered me down and tried again, this time succeeding in manoeuvring me into a chair. Once sitting I immediately become hot and dizzy. I could not cope with the change in position, my head suddenly upright after spending so long lying flat, and I threw up green bile.

Just before my injury, Nathan and I had been watching *Twin Peaks*. After the villain, Leo, is shot and sustains a brain injury, he is left in the care of his ex-girlfriend and her new partner. There is a scene where an eccentric hoist seller comes to their house. As Leo dangles from an exaggeratedly tall machine, he is swung around the room and crashes into the walls; a slapstick horror show. Suddenly it felt painfully close to home.

I was learning quickly that I would have to advocate hard, even for basic needs. I felt completely at the whim of others, not only as a patient but a newly disabled one. The number of times I had to call my mum, crying, to ask her to call the front desk of the ward so someone would come and open the door and give me back the call button that had been left just out of reach.

'Why are you so tired today, Grace?' staff would ask me brightly most mornings. How exhausting it was. It was a tiredness I had never experienced and have not experienced since. I felt as though I was being hollowed out.

Early on, I nearly choked on an ibuprofen. I was taking my breakfast assortment of blue, white and pink pills from the paper pot. I picked up the thick, pastel pink ibuprofen, nearly the size of a 5p coin. I tried to swallow it, but it became lodged in my throat.

I tried to gesture frantically at Nathan and my dad, but they were distracted, chatting by the window. My abdominal muscles now flaccid and uncooperative, I couldn't summon any strength to cough it up. For a second, while it was stuck, I thought about the irony of it all. I had survived a man jumping on to me from a height of thirty metres but I was going to die a week later from choking on an ibuprofen tablet. Luckily, with enough effort, I swallowed it down.

My nurse at the time responded by liquefying all my tablets from then on. The worst of it by far, though, was that she kept trying to persuade me that this assortment of chalky liquids would taste nice. Even the senna tablet, a laxative made from what looks (and tastes) like dehydrated mud, was liquidised. She pressed these on me: 'No, they'll be yummy!' she would coo, as if feeding a baby.

Sometimes I felt as though I had been left to rot in that bed, waiting to be seen, chasing up scans and updates on plans. After many requests, I finally got a physiotherapist to come down and see me.

A man strode in first, a junior following. They asked me what I could move so far, and I said nothing. They assessed my range of motion by bending, straightening and rotating my thin, floppy legs. While the male physiotherapist held my inanimate right leg in the air, talking about my risks of pressure sores, he looked down at me:

'Don't worry, soon your skin will become leathery and will be used to it.' He smiled confidently.

I said thanks, stunned that 'leathery' was the word he'd chosen, as if that was supposed to comfort me.

But, although the level of indignity in those weeks

was often vast, and the bruising humiliations regular, I was shown so much kindness, too. And as we got into the swing of physio, there were breakthroughs small and large; many times I felt like a newborn baby learning every milestone again for the first time. Sometimes it felt like my heart had never been so full.

Being a patient often means being in a highly fragile, highly dynamic state. It was for me.

It was a time I had never felt more vulnerable, but also a time I had never felt more loved. After my injury I experienced what I can only describe as the closest thing to my funeral. The way people spoke to me, sent me cards, writing about moments from our shared past, some I had forgotten. Seeing some be vulnerable, crying in front of me, surprised me. I saw sides of people I hadn't been witness to before.

Friends would congregate on the hospital's fourth-floor café each day, resorting to arts and crafts to pass the time. These artworks of varying quality would get sent up to me on the eleventh floor to judge.

I was also buoyed by late-night conversations with nurses and healthcare assistants while they cleaned and dressed me when I couldn't do it for myself. Some days I wrote down their names, and it's funny looking at them now because I have no idea who *Stella* and *Charice* are. They must have felt so important to me at the time.

There is a photo of me from those early days smiling as I sipped wonton soup. My neck brace meant that I couldn't bend my neck properly to drink so Nathan had constructed an elongated straw out of three straws so I could reach the soup.

I clung on to these small pieces of joy.

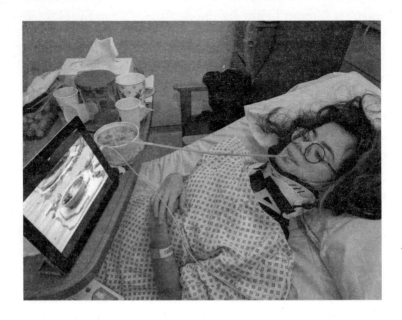

It's hard to recall all the painful moments I experienced in what would stretch into three months as a patient, but the damage has been long-lasting. There was neither time nor space to grieve in hospital. At times it felt like my pain had nowhere to go. When I was eventually discharged, it felt as though I was returning from a war that only I had fought.

Medical trauma is a tricky creature, and I have told very few people about mine.

It's something that would come back to haunt me

when I found myself on the other side. Pieces of me were taken away after every invasive test, every assessment. After every indignity. Many may well have been necessary but all the same, awful. So often I felt as though I wasn't a human being any more.

I have no residual traumatic memories from that day in Westfield; I hardly remember it. But the hours, days, weeks and months that followed, when my body was passed over and over, when I felt I was in control of nothing, left a lasting impact.

As determined as I was to recover, to wake up every day, there was a horror in all of it that I couldn't fully comprehend until I left hospital. It's a horror that took me years to process, and I still find myself flinching, closing up, freezing when touched at times. It has taken me years to get over.

I am aware that, in medicine, we must do some inevitably uncomfortable, inevitably painful things to patients every day, but we must be able to do this without victimising them at the same time, so people can leave with their sense of self intact. That is our purpose. To make the horrifying as bearable as possible.

It has made me determined to protect the dignity of my own patients, in any way I can.

Before

25 October 2018

Damien, my designated police officer, is sitting opposite my hospital bed. It is odd to think I have a designated anything, and with the word designated I imagine he should be pocket-sized, so that I can carry him around and bring him out for all my police officer needs. An earnest man, overly polite, he looks out of place in his ironed shirt sitting on this plastic NHS chair in front of me.

I've noticed that since being here, in this state, people tend to shrink when faced with me. I think of how unwell I must look.

He has come to film my victim impact statement, another strange and foreign term. I am bewildered by it.

His colleague, a similarly earnest man in a white shirt, has set up a film camera pointed at me, while Damien asks the first question.

'What were you like before your injury?'

He holds a pen and notebook, poised to take down my answer. It's not one of those detective notepads, where you flip over the pages and jot down clues like 'screwdriver found at the scene' or 'she was wearing a blue cardigan'. There is no investigation needed, no mystery to what occurred last week, it is solid fact. Apparently.

I am struggling to understand his use of this word, before.

What was I like before? This *thing* had only just happened, and I found it hard to acknowledge that there was suddenly a before and an after, and I was now firmly in the *after*. That I could not go back.

The question suggested it was obvious I will not be like I was; that time is over, when it felt like it was only just beginning.

I was only twenty-two. I was not yet formed. I felt like sculpted sand that could disappear in the waves.

I could not qualify the 'I' in that moment. It was much easier to think of myself in relation to others. Who are we if not made up of the people we love?

I looked past Damien to my mother and father, who were anxiously looking back at me, their only child. I felt a pang of guilt ; I had given them enough to worry about in my short time on earth already.

Beginning with my premature birth, which had nearly killed me and my mother in the process, when her blood pressure became unmanageable, and I was pulled out tiny and desperately in need of blood. Born with so few red cells, the doctors went through a long list of diagnoses. Did I have leukaemia? Or something else? As the scant blood cells I did have plummeted, it took months for doctors to discover I had something so rare many hadn't even heard of it: Diamond-Blackfan anaemia. In medical school I would find it was a single sentence in a textbook. After three gifts of blood from strangers, I was pushed into remission when I was less than a year old.

I thought then of myself aged seven visiting my Australian family, playing an elaborate game of 'touch the end of the boat ramp and run back before the wave hits you', under the bad influence of my older cousin. Of course, I was not fast enough running back along the volcanic rocks, and the Tasmanian winter sea swallowed me up. I sank, hand still gripped tightly to the plastic hand of my Baby Born doll. My mother dived in to grab me without question before my head could go under.

I thought of a few years later when I stepped on a sea urchin clinging to the rocks where we went on holiday every year in Turkey and walked back through the mud, my bright yellow crocs offering poor protection. That night I woke up screaming in pain, a red line from my foot that foreshadowed sepsis beginning to inch up my calf through my lymph system. My parents drove through the night to the nearest village where I was given giant green tablets at the tiny hospital, and the red line recoiled before it could make its way to my heart.

But I had never come closer to death than I did in here, a few days ago.

How many chances do I get at a life? This felt like a lot already.

But I come from strong stock. Growing up we were an impenetrable family unit, my parents and I, a house of stability for others to find respite in. As an only child I spent nearly all my time with them and their friends;

babysitters were a foreign concept to me. I can see why only children are considered a peculiar breed to those with larger families. There is something so very intense about it. It's hard to describe my childhood, but it is sacred to me, and I am the only keeper of it.

We spent every summer in Turkey in a small town by the sea with my adopted grandmother, Hacer. She is family not through blood, but through my mother walking into an antique store in Istanbul one day thirty years ago and starting a conversation, leading to a decades-long friendship. It's funny how the smallest choices can create vast waves. She is formidable, a force. It's hard to believe she was ever anything other than who she is now. I imagine her always as fully formed.

Curling up in my dad's lap in his fleece jacket, listening to Hacer speak Turkish, was a large part of my childhood. It is a rich, velvety language. Sometimes I wish I could bottle up her turns of phrase, the way she says certain words, like unbeLIEVable. The lilts and cracks in her voice.

The bungalow where we stayed was a seven-hour drive from Istanbul airport, and one holiday we arrived late one night to find the whole place flooded and without electricity. We lit candles and all climbed into my parents' bed, eating bread and cheese cross-legged in the dark. Protected from the two centimetres of water on the floor, but we could have been floating on the Aegean Sea for all I cared. Everyone I needed was sitting on that mattress.

My sun-freckled, beautiful parents.

They had met in Launceston, Australia, a small town on the island of Tasmania, where everyone knows everyone.

My paternal grandfather, at one point the town's only paediatrician, and maternal grandmother, a paediatric physiotherapist, worked together. Launceston feels a little like a toy town. Red-roofed houses, coloured walls, neat front gardens and porches, local shops selling sweets and meat pies. It is made up of a collection of hills, and my two grandmothers lived on one each, which meant you could look out over all the little houses through each of their garden windows. It is a place where everyone is known by their family name, or by some nickname picked up thirty years before. A place that seems to have an inordinate number of freak accidents and tragedies, likely because everyone is about two points of contact away from each other, and news travels fast.

I was sure half of Tasmania knew what had happened to me already, halfway around the world.

My mother is a professor of state crime, who has made it her life's work to document injustice. My father is a soft-spoken, calm, collected, organised professor in string theory. The things that he could create in his head with a blank piece of paper will always amaze me. There was, unfortunately (or fortunately), not much need, in Tasmania, for research into string theory or genocide, so they had moved to England for work, settling in London in the eighties. Living as a Tasmanian Londoner I feel like an oxymoron, straddling two very different places without feeling completely settled in one or the other. It sometimes leaves me feeling as though I don't have proper roots in either.

*

I thought about my partner, Nathan, who had at that moment just gone out to get me a pastry, most likely from the coffee shop adjacent to the hospital where he racked up extortionate bills, returning with handfuls of overpriced treats every time. He would bring me the sun if he thought it would make me smile.

His way of coping with what had happened had been to sit by my bedside every minute he could, much to the irritation of the ward matron. Years later I see she had documented exasperated conversations with him about infection control. But he was undeterred. He gave me the absolute certainty that we were dealing with this together.

He is a green-eyed, brown-haired boy who walked up to me in our university library when I was in second year and asked, 'Don't I know you from somewhere?'

I was pretty sure he didn't, but I liked the approach.

He was a physics student; the next time I saw him I was on the bus on my way to hockey practice, and he was scribbling equations in his notebook. I had grown up in a house full of such scribbles.

He was so unlike me in many ways, which came as a relief. He was calm, I was at times neurotic; he was analytical, and I jumped in with feelings. He hung all his socks up in colour order on the radiator by his bed. He loved music and books and got excited when talking about something he liked.

On our first date we drank red wine from a box and watched *High Fidelity*. I leant my head on his shoulder that night, and it felt like I had arrived home. I spent that summer riding around Peckham on the back of his bicycle. I started writing poetry again, about his green eyes and the planes flying over as we lay in his room, just large enough to fit a double bed. Young and in love.

We moved on to a boat together by Tower Bridge connected to twenty other barges, with a garden of flowers growing on top of each one. There were some less than romantic things about that place I'd have to admit; living with four others (including a ketamine addict) and emptying the toilet waste tank with a suction tube every week, for starters.

But it still felt like a dream to live there, stepping on to the bridge from the street, pulling the wooden trap door into our cosy barge that had a wood-burning stove. I loved watching the sun go down on the ducks with my legs dangling over the edge. Being rocked to sleep every night.

I thought of the room we had just decorated, the first place we had lived together. The carpets, the musty smell, the plants, the books, the brass porthole window that had just been replaced. The wooden clothes chest I had painted blue. I couldn't yet think about what would happen to that boat. That I had left it one day and would now never return.

I thought of Juan, my old climbing coach, who had come to visit me just before the police interview.

I first met Juan when I was thirteen. I was thrilled to have got into the illustrious competition squad at the Castle Climbing Centre, a step up from the kids' club where I had trained for the previous five years. The Castle is an old Victorian waterworks building converted into a climbing gym, and since visiting aged seven it had rapidly become my second home.

A tough, tattooed Venezuelan man, Juan took no bullshit. I was a little scared of him at first. We started calling his intense pep talks 'Juan to ones' and I soon learned that all he really wanted was for us to succeed. He is one of the few people I can rely on to always be brutally honest with me.

Before I got into climbing, I had always felt a bit left behind. My premature birth and anaemia meant I was dangerously close to dropping off the weight and height charts for my age, so much so that my doctor had to put me on a 'chocolate mousse diet'. People always assumed I was younger than I was because of my size. But I was desperate to be helpful, and furious when the boys were asked to help carry boxes in primary school and I wasn't.

I never felt as hardy or tough as my older Australian cousins. I would get cold easily and was so sensitive to my environment, or to any slight. Returning to Australia for holidays every two years, I was always back to being the youngest, the weakest.

The one thing that made me feel capable was climbing. I was never an athletic child, but I loved to clamber over rocks, fit into small spaces, swing from tree branches. I was *good* at this, and it was so exciting. I would train every day, hanging from a bar above my bedroom, creating intricate training plans in preparation for competitions. I would try a climb again, and again, and again, until I was bleeding and crying, tears and sweat running down my face.

It made me feel brave, capable and, combined with

my eagerness to please and overcompensate for my tiny frame, it gave me the courage to always put my hand up, to volunteer to be first.

I had started working as a coach at the Castle to cover my boat rent and Juan had become my mentor. I appreciated his coming to visit even more after he told me his dad had passed away on this same ward, a bay over. I knew he had been hit by a bus and had spent six months in a coma before his death, but I hadn't realised it was right here, where I found myself.

Juan had brought me fancy chocolates and resistance bands, along with a list of exercises to start trying. He winked at me as he gave me the chocolates, one of which had a small pipette of rum you squirted into it.

He held the resistance band up high and I pulled down.

'Keep the elbow closer to you, Gracie girl . . . for now your left is a little weaker than your right.'

It felt like we were back at the climbing wall: I was thirteen and he was coaching me again. He was not giving up on me.

'Breathe, Gracie girl, just breathe.'

I thought of my friends from university sitting in the hospital canteen three floors down, anxiously awaiting any news. I was a fourth year in medical school and felt as though I was finally finding my stride.

I had received four rejections before being accepted into one university, after an interview in which the doctors were thankfully more interested in hearing about my recent climbing competition and didn't mind that I didn't know the four principles of medical ethics very well.

I will be forever grateful to those two older men sitting in armchairs, willing to give me a chance. It felt like months after everyone else had received their acceptances, but I was thrilled.

The first year had been a tidal wave of knowledge, facts, elaborate Latin terms. I always felt behind in those hours spent drawing and redrawing chemical pathways, our supervisor intent on us being able to recite every amino acid by heart. I was terrible at histology and dreaded those Thursday mornings spent peering down microscopes at squiggly red blood cells in archaic oak-panelled rooms.

I had always loved learning and working hard, but I struggled at university, living away from home for the first time. I was suddenly so below average. I earned the nickname '38' briefly for getting 38 per cent in the mathematics quiz. How could other people seem to manage it all? I would draw life-size pictures of the human body, willing it to go into my head, but I still didn't know the mesentery from the omentum.

Unsurprisingly, I failed every gruelling exam I took in first year, and spent that summer locked in my bedroom at my parents' house furiously revising, having to confront the possibility that I wasn't cut out for this. I remember naively thinking I would rather lose a limb than lose my place.

Thankfully I passed my resits and was much more capable once the people side of things began. Hospital placements as a medical student sometimes made you feel less useful than the bin you were hovering next to, but I loved them all the same.

I took a year out of medicine to do a master's at the London School of Hygiene and Tropical Medicine, a magical-looking building tucked behind the British Museum, a stone banner around its perimeter engraved with the names of health pioneers, steps leading up to a gold and marble front door. We had classes on what creates health inequalities, how to make an impact sustainable, and the influence of corporations like the tobacco and alcohol industry.

It felt bigger than anything I had learned before: political, exciting, important.

Nathan had just started a PhD in physics, and it seemed like we were both growing into ourselves.

The summer before I went back to medical school I took a trip to Palestine, the first time I had travelled on my own, doing research for my dissertation. I was terrified, interviewing strangers in remote places that I'd take two buses through armed checkpoints to get to, but I managed it.

It was the 2018 World Cup, and I remember they played it on a projector in the courtyard of the Jerusalem hotel. Clutching a drink ticket I had been given on arrival I asked for a beer, and for the first time sat on my own in a restaurant. I went climbing in Ramallah with people I'd just met and remember turning around to hear the call to prayer while hanging off a mountain. I felt good, strong and excited about what was to come.

I had survived that trip on my own. I was still so

young, but I felt on the precipice, becoming more confident, capable, adventurous. I was filling out the outlines
of myself.

Overnight I had woken up in a body that did not feel like
my own. What little sense of self I had had been scraped
clean, bled dry.

Who would I be to all these people now?

I was yanked from my youth, pulled back from the
path I had begun to forge for myself. Now there was a
void, and suddenly I was scrabbling, slipping down a
crevasse, clutching at crumbling handholds.

The hospital, a place I had been so comfortable in just
the day before, where I had been learning and growing,
the place of my future, had become my hell for the next
three months.

Patient

PSYCH REFERRAL

Patient was admitted when a person jumped from a balcony and landed on her - she is now paraplegic and trying to deal with this life-changing diagnosis. No suicidal thoughts expressed.

Patient was in bed awake and alert, she consented for assessment to take place.

Patient reported feeling like she should talk to someone about what happened to her. Patient denied any rumination related to the incident or the perpetrator.

She struggles to be assertive with her healthcare. She reported numerous episodes of being left in the room, door closed, alone without her call bell. She also reported some staff talking to her about religion and 'God's will' despite her being atheist. She also reported some difficulty in telling visitors to leave when she needs a break.

Patient continues to be future-focused, goal-oriented and realistic about the future and occupied. She is sleeping well. Good appetite.

Impression: Normal adjustment

Ten days into my hospital stay and the neck brace I had to wear following the surgery was slowly driving me to despair. It was way too big for me, and the plastic edge of it dug into my jaw. A gnawing, constant pain.

As the surgeons had decided not to bolt the fracture in place, they were hoping bone would heal around the break if kept stiffly in the same position by the brace.

I asked one of the doctors if I could try a smaller one, one that might fit me better, and he promised he would investigate.

A while later, a man in the short-sleeved white shirt of a physiotherapist strolled in, unannounced.

'Hello,' he said as he wandered around the room.

I didn't like his casual attitude, the way he sauntered in, without introducing himself.

'Hello, who are you?' I replied.

He looked taken aback by this question and laughed. He wasn't used to being spoken to like that by a patient, he said.

He bent down next to my bed, smiled and stared at me, tilting his head to the side as he asked, 'Why do you think you *need* a neck brace?'

I knew this question well; we were taught to use it as a tool to assess if a patient understands the severity of their own situation, but here it felt so condescending. I was furious. He thinks I am oblivious to what has happened to me, and that my answer is going to confirm this.

'I have a Jefferson fracture of my C1 vertebra,' I replied curtly. I was glad I remembered that.

Did he think I couldn't appreciate how serious this was? I was painfully aware that my head currently sat on broken bones, how necessary this brace was, but why must any patient go through this test, this humiliation, just to get a collar that actually fits? I couldn't quite see what I needed to prove, just because I had asked for a different size.

I had learned about the top neck bones in my second year of medical school, hours spent trying to get my head around the blood and nerve supply that wove in and out of those bony orifices. Roots becoming trunks, cords, divisions, leading to tiny delicate branches running down the shoulders.

The atlas bone, also known as C1, is the first vertebra of the neck, on which sits the skull. The axis bone is the second, C2, which has a rounded bump called the odontoid process that fits snugly into the atlas bone. Holding them in dissection class, I remember how satisfying it was putting them together, marvelling at nature's ability to create perfectly fitting pieces.

I have read that a Jefferson fracture is a fracture of the thin back arches of that C1 bone, arches which hug my spinal cord. I couldn't help imagining those tiny fractures giving way, more shards of bone plunging into nerves.

I realised early on after my injury that I had a certain burden of knowledge, and I couldn't decide if that was a good or bad thing. If it was helping or harming me in that moment.

*

After finding the first few years of medical school so difficult, I was just starting to get into the swing of things when this happened. Bar a short obsession aged five with delivering pizzas, medicine was the only thing I had ever wanted to do. I had grown up feeling at home in hospitals, visiting the friendly paediatricians every year to ensure my blood condition continued to be in remission.

Other than nearly dying at birth, I had been very lucky. I was 'the most well person with the condition' that my haematologist had ever seen. Diamond-Blackfan anaemia became nothing more than an interesting collection of words, a fun fact to share about myself. I had been saved, and I think I understood that from an early age.

Recently I had a blood test, and the particular smell of an alcohol wipe and the feel of a fabric tourniquet wrapped around my arm like the ones used when I was a child struck me with a nostalgia so strong that I thought I would cry. It brought back so vividly the feeling of being looked after.

I was not a calm child. Perpetually anxious, in fact. I hated the time just before going to sleep, alone with my thoughts. The prospect of being the last one awake at a sleepover filled me with dread. But a hospital is always awake, always humming with activity; and that was comforting to me. Perhaps that was why I was so drawn to them.

Growing up, I compulsively read a battered copy of the British Medical Association's 1997 *Children's Symptoms: The Quick Reference Guide to Identification and Treatment, Including Essential First Aid*. It had a fittingly nineties cover: photographs of children looking unwell, framed with bright red and blue borders. Bought by my conscientious parents in preparation for their first and only child, every page had flowcharts of different symptoms that would eventually lead to a diagnosis.

START HERE: *Does your child have any of the following symptoms?*

Fever, seems unwell, sneezing, runny nose, coughing, none of the above.

Aged seven I would go through each chart, choosing what symptoms I could have that day, tracing my finger along the arrows, wanting to know what it would lead to. What could I be diagnosed with next? Diabetes? Meningitis? Head injury? Substance abuse? Poisoning? Glue ear? Febrile convulsions?

It excited me, this journey to discovery. It all seemed so clear, so neat, that you could compile these problems into categories to help people. You find a problem, you fix it.

The early years of medical school reinforced these straightforward ideas of health and sickness. The first two years consisted mainly of lectures and small group classes. We started on a cellular level, looking through microscopes at purple- and red-stained blobs. It was important to have this base of knowledge, but the behaviour of cells felt far removed from a real patient presenting with a real problem, which seemed a terrifying prospect.

As a first-year medical student, I encountered a dead body long before I saw a living patient. In groups of seven we spent a year with an allocated cadaver, his face covered with a sheet, as the second-year students did head and neck dissection simultaneously. I nearly passed out the first time I entered that hot and heavy room.

I tried to memorise the bones and muscles and their attachments, but never knew the correct answer when they would pull an unidentified piece from the body. It was hard to concentrate when the smell of formaldehyde used to preserve the cadavers made me feel simultaneously faint and starving. My best friend and I would hold the cadaver's ankles while our other classmates dissected the pelvis and muscles of the legs. 'Holding the ankles' became a symbol for how I spent that first year; watching from the end of the bed as others got stuck in.

I didn't think much about disability back then, or where it might sit in my binary notions of who was well or unwell; I didn't have to. I may have been studying disease and disability, but I lived in a very able world. What we were taught was almost always based on the white, able male body; everyone else felt like the exception.

The one teaching session around disability that I do remember was a workshop with a blind man and his personal assistant. We sat in a circle and listened, as his assistant spoke over him multiple times. We were taught how to help lead him into the clinic room by bending an elbow so he could hook his hand in the crook of our arm. Did we learn anything else? About how he navigated life outside of this room, and the barriers he faced? About his priorities, his values, his concerns?

Sure, I could guide him into a room, but what would happen next?

This epitomised my teaching on disability; it was

confined to the clinic room, with no context given around the real-life experiences of a disabled person. I never questioned this 'medical' approach to disability, where it is individualised and pathologised. A problem to be fixed. The underlying message was always that it was the specific injury or impairment that disabled someone, rather than their environment, social context or the political climate.

This was the model that presided when I was a student and continues to preside in medicine today. After all, if the foundations of modern medicine are based on keeping the army-aged, able-bodied male fighting fit, how could disability be seen as anything other than a failure of that same medicine?

It reminded me starkly of how I had felt at sixteen when my mother and climbing coach had noticed my posture was quite poor. I was seen by an orthopaedic doctor and told that I had a kyphosis, a curvature of the spine. I spent hours doing exercises to straighten my back, wearing a brace, walking back and forth in a straight line while a physiotherapist critiqued my form. The aversion, the shame I felt.

I sat in an appointment in the outpatient clinic many months and exercises later, crying to the doctor as he showed me my scan. We analysed my vertebral wedge angles on the X-ray, down the corridor from the very same ward I would become painfully familiar with when my spine was crushed years later. It's laughable: wedge angles would become the least of my problems, but at the time, to me, this was the worst possible thing. I must be faultless, and if I had a fault, it was up to me to fix it.

As a teenager I was already experiencing the shame that came with being faced with an ideal I could not match, a measurement I could not reach. The tyranny of perfectionism, the desperation to fit in.

Soon after my injury I was reduced to a series of numbers and letters: T4 incomplete SCI; ASIA (American Spinal Injury Association Impairment scale) score B. My spinal cord was injured at the fourth thoracic vertebra – T4 – and the letter B indicated that I had sensation but no movement below the level of my injury.

This was following an assessment made by a physiotherapist to determine my baseline. I would have a few of these assessments throughout the weeks as an inpatient to gauge if there had been any improvement. He arrived at my bed armed with cotton wool, a sharp pin and a tuning fork, a strange array of equipment that would determine my score. This was another test I could not prepare myself for.

I would soon learn that every part of me, every activity I did, every bodily function would be given a numerical value.

A is for 'Complete', which has a slightly contentious definition, depending on who you speak to. You can take it to mean the spinal cord has been completely severed; or that there is no sensation or movement below the 'level' of the injury (where the spinal cord has been damaged).

'Incomplete' covers both B, for some sensation, and C, for some sensation and some movement below the injury level.

The categories for sensation are pinprick, dull, light touch and vibration. As if a category could document the nature of touch that I now feel. How do I describe the ripples of vibration flowing down the sides of my knees and parts of my legs when I'm in the shower? What category denotes that the outlines of my feet are clear, while in other places there is a complete absence, as if those parts of me don't exist any more. That I can be sure where my legs are in space, only to look down and realise I've got it all wrong. That every one of my nerve endings feels burnt. That electricity rushes through my legs and meets these fried ends and with nowhere to go produces an endless static, as if I am constantly buzzing.

He tested every area of my skin according to a nerve map. I've loved this map since we learned about it in second year. It is so neat; each nerve root branches out from the spinal cord into smaller and smaller branches, supplying a clearly demarcated area of skin.

My map had been scribbled on; parts rubbed out.

For months, I held on tightly to these numbers and letters I was given. As if they were a passport to my new self. I was suddenly categorised, but at the same time felt I could not fit myself into these strict definitions. They were too crude, too one-dimensional. I was finding there was little room for my reality within them.

Before my injury I had just finished my last week of women's health and was about to begin four months on long-term conditions, which included a placement in geriatrics. I had recently learned of the frailty score, a rating system used in hospitals to assess older adults. It can be used to determine if someone is suitable for a life-saving operation, or to predict their prognosis. The template begins with a black and white image of a strong, fit man; as you move along the scale, mobility devices appear like omens. There is only one wheelchair on the page, illustrating the last point:

LIVING WITH SEVERE FRAILTY: completely dependent for personal care, from whatever cause (physical or cognitive). Even so, they seem stable and not at high risk of dying (within 6 months).

I understand this is for over 65-year-olds, but will I be dismissed as I get older? Where will I be placed? Where could I find myself? I do not fit anywhere in this diagram. I am not considered. Like trying to jam a square peg into a round hole. A seated person into a standing outline.

In many ways I could not superimpose myself on to anything I had learned in medical school. I was no longer on the bell curve, but an aberrant point, or rather not on the graph at all.

None of this felt right. I realised how inadequate my previous attitudes and preconceptions had been, faced with the reality of living as a disabled person.

PART 2:
Rehabilitation

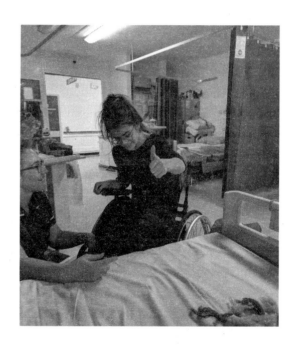

Stanmore

SNAPS II – *Stanmore nursing assessment of psychological rating sheet*

Patient name: Grace Spence Green

Positive motivation
  0 = is positively motivated

Fear, anxiety
  1 = seems tense and preoccupied much of the time

Sadness
  1 = appears quite sad, sometimes tearful
  Patient seen crying after partner and parents left

Burden
  0 = not duly concerned about burdening others

Relationships with family
  0 = generally good family relationships
  Family with her until quite late as first day on unit

Relationships with staff
  0 = generally good relationships with staff

Irritability/hostility/ anger
  0 = seems generally to be at peace with self and others

Withdrawal/ isolation/disengagement
  0 = mixes frequently with others

A volunteer from one of the spinal injury charities came to visit me a few days after my conversation with my surgeon.

I was taken aback when she wheeled in, manoeuvring the biggest power chair I had ever seen. It was raised off the floor, so she towered over everyone. She was wearing a blazer and silver skirt, which matched the silver streak in her hair. She had a large silver handbag hooked around her elbow, from which she brought out an iPad to tap in my details.

I was curious about the way she moved, the way she typed. It was as though I was seeing a disabled person clearly for the first time. Her hands were folded into fists, and she used her wrists to manoeuvre her bag around her lap.

I was to go on outdoor courses, wheelchair skills classes, and sit-ski trips in Colorado she explained, while quickly typing on her iPad with her knuckles. I was in a new club now: one that I don't remember getting the invitation to, and wasn't sure if I wanted to be part of it.

But first, before the skiing, I needed to go to the Royal National Orthopaedic Hospital in Stanmore, a specialist rehabilitation centre on the northern outskirts of London.

Soon after this visit, I was strapped to a gurney, bundled into an ambulance and shipped off to Stanmore.

It was not the countryside manor that I had, perhaps naively, pictured. Built in the 1920s, it's a ramshackle collection of buildings that connect via ramps and outhouses. It looked a bit like a bungalow whose over-zealous owner had a penchant for DIY, adding extensions in odd places so that it splayed out in different directions, a spider with ill-proportioned limbs.

During my time as a patient there, a brand-new hospital on the same site was under construction, giving it an even more unfinished appearance. In the grey of November, it was particularly bleak.

The hospital's spinal unit had been opened by the Princess of Wales in the eighties, and it didn't look like much had been updated since then.

All around me were newly injured people who had arrived here for many different reasons. They had fallen off balconies, crashed every type of vehicle possible, dived into shallow water, tripped over concrete paving. They had tumours or bone pressing on their spinal cord, tuberculosis or their own immune system attacking their nervous system and were all at different levels of injury with varying degrees of function and movement.

I was no longer alone in this plight, for better or worse.

The weekend before my injury, friends and I had found an empty field near our residence in Maidstone, got drunk and had a bonfire. We laughed around the rough fire we had made, giggling, sharing ghost stories, holding hands and stumbling our way out of the field. I stayed up all night to watch the sunrise with my best friend.

Now I find I have lost control of every bodily function, in a place I cannot leave.

*

There were only three other female patients in the spinal unit, and so we made up the one female bay of four beds. The other women were all above fifty, and I didn't feel as though we had a lot in common. The first thing that Edith, the lady in the bed opposite me, told me was that she watched the CCTV of my injury on BBC news, and joked I was infamous and that she should get my autograph.

It was not a great start.

Then I was introduced to my consultant, Dr Wood. A sharp, cold woman with a razor-cut black fringe, who would come around every Monday morning to glance at me and my lack of 'development'.

I had a case manager, who was in charge of helping me navigate the mountain of paperwork and admin that was waiting for me now that I belong to a different category in society. I soon found our conversations so draining that I would duck out of corridors just to avoid him.

I also had an army of physiotherapists, occupational therapists, nurses, other doctors, healthcare assistants and wheelchair technicians.

I was here to be *rehabilitated*, whatever that meant. Brought back to being a functioning member of society.

I will be fixed here, repackaged as new. This would all be a small blip in my otherwise straightforward life. I don't belong here; this isn't part of my plan. My brain kept falling back on these thoughts, but the evidence was there in my motionless legs. How many times did I have to remind myself that this *had* happened. That I was no longer temporarily 'sick', with a set time span for recovery. I wasn't confined to bed any more like in the Royal London, eating takeaway and watching Netflix.

Here, I had to be up every day, learning to interact with my body in ways I had never had to before – and quickly.

I was exactly where I needed to be.

When does denial become a kind of self-hatred? I was not only denying my current reality, I was denying my new future.

12 November 2018

The first morning, I am given a big bright blue folder to read and a timetable for the week to come. Every day I would be doing occupational therapy and physiotherapy.

The folder has coloured diagrams of spinal cords, explaining how nerves control our sensation and movement. There are chapters and tests on nutrition, breathing, pressure sores, and other topics that now seem very important to my new life. I couldn't remember learning much about spinal cord injuries in medical school. Just one of many slides I must have glanced over. I am desperate to learn now, to tick the boxes, to move forward.

Fran, my assigned occupational therapist, whose no-nonsense attitude is a balm to my fluctuating emotions, gets me out of bed and into a wheelchair by the second day of my stay.

She teaches me to use my knuckles to lift myself on to a wooden board that bridges between the bed and the wheelchair cushion. She tells me to put my left fist on the bed close to my left hip, and my right fist on to the wheelchair cushion, to direct where I want to end up. I then lift and shift my body weight around. I land in the wheelchair, just about.

It doesn't feel like I have a centre of balance any more, I am not used to the new dynamics of my body. I fall forward on to my knees trying to wheel my way to the break room.

I was thrown into wheelchair skills lessons; I soon learned how to lean and balance on my back wheels, how to manoeuvre corners, pushing up and rolling down the dangerously steep corridor that ran the length of the hospital, named the 'San Francisco slope' by staff. So steep that they had to use electric stair climber machines to drag the hospital beds up from the operating theatre at the bottom.

I hated the wheelchair, but I reluctantly went to the classes.

My group included the only other person under the age of forty on my ward, Rubes, who had crashed his quad bike in Croatia and whose acceptance and grace I envied; and Brian, a middle-aged man whose special skill was squirting water through the large gap between his front teeth at unsuspecting patients like me. The first time I met Brian we played catch in the gym as a balancing exercise, throwing a heavy ball to one another, each of us sitting cross-legged on opposite plinths. Every so often one of us would fall backwards with the impact of the ball, and lie on our back like a beetle, not yet able to right ourselves without help.

We didn't make the ideal team to teach; Brian didn't like to follow instructions and Rubes could be over-zealous, once managing to tip out of his wheelchair in the gym. And me? I alternated between determination and hopelessness.

As the weeks went on, however, Brian developed a permanent scowl on his face. He stopped coming to physio and our wheelchair skills classes. I would often find him lying on the sofa in the day room with a jumper over his face. He, like a handful of the other patients, had checked out of the process. As if not trying in this reality would deny the truth of it.

It was hard to be in a place where everyone around me was struggling. We were all going through such acute stages of grief.

Every patient in the unit was allocated a psychologist that they saw weekly. I was given a psychiatrist; perhaps, having read about the out of the ordinary circumstances surrounding my injury, they believed I might need someone able to prescribe me something.

I warmed to him, and we talked about how to deal with this new grief. I hadn't thought of it in those terms before. He described my brain as a big box with a 'pain' button on one side, and inside the box was a ball bouncing around, hitting the walls. Every time it hit the pain button it would make me wince. At that moment, he would tell me, my ball was huge, but it would get smaller, and these visceral pangs would become less frequent, less intense.

Back then it felt as though this ball engulfed everything I thought, everything I did, everyone I was with. I couldn't imagine ever getting out from under the shade it cast.

Stanmore was an initiation into the new ways I had to learn to manage what comes out of me. The staff taught me quickly, brutally. There was no time to feel unhappy about it. To grieve my old, much less complicated life.

I was given 'magic bullets', suppositories made of sugar that irritate the bowel lining. I learned to insert them myself to give my body a new signal that it's time to go to the bathroom, bypassing the spinal cord. I must do this at a similar time every day.

My indwelling, or long-term, catheter was removed, and I was taught to insert and remove a tube myself, a single-use catheter. I had no idea where to aim the first time, and so two nurses watched on as I prodded and poked myself until finally, exhausted and sore, pee eventually came out.

I was told I would need to do this every four hours for the rest of my life.

I was taught to measure and record my urine output in volumes every time at first: phone notes I find later filled with meaningless numbers.

I was given a new rule book for my body to follow. Routine. Routine. Routine. It was drilled into me that I must never deviate from the routine.

In some ways it was much harder to become accustomed to this than to using a wheelchair. I felt completely alone. I knew no one else who did any of this.

*

The bathroom became a place of pain, but also of peace. Where I would throw up every day for the first two weeks while sitting on the toilet, my head unable to cope with being so suddenly upright every morning after weeks lying flat. And yet it was the only place where I could be alone. The place I could finally shower after five weeks of bed baths. I grinned all the way through my first shower, vowing to never take this absolute miracle for granted again.

The shower was a huge respite. As a child, I used to sit cross-legged on the bathroom floor by the heat of the radiator, wrapped in a towel, watching water drip from my hair and make patterns on the mat. I would remember how, when I was little, my father would wrap me in a towel after I'd had a bath and pretend I was a parcel going to be delivered to the Post Office.

It was my only safe, quiet place on the ward.

I began to talk to my legs in the shower. As challenging as it all was, I felt like I was loving and caring for my body more than I ever did before. I wanted to look after it. It needed help. Now, to clean my toes, I have to lean down to grab my foot and pull it over on to my other leg. The water doesn't feel like water; instead I feel only vibrations around the sides of my knees, my feet, my ankles, the left-hand side of my stomach and the backs of my thighs.

After learning some basic wheelchair skills and getting my bladder and bowel under some control, I began to be reintegrated into the public: learning to drive in the hospital car park, and a supervised visit to a nearby pub for lunch. I was taken to the pub in a van, anchored down to the floor and wearing a foam neck brace. Strapped in there and back for an allocated two-hour visit outside, it was hard not to feel like a prisoner out on day release. Particularly when the irritable driving instructor had accidentally referred to me as a 'disabled inmate' in our first lesson.

This will end. This will end. This will end. I told myself over and over.

My parents and Nathan did the three-hour return drive every day to visit me. They brought home-cooked food and huddled around my hospital bed to watch films. They too were going through something vast, but they were the ropes that kept me anchored.

As much as I despised Stanmore and the unbearable greyness of it all, it was the first place I experienced a certain kind of kinship. One that I would cherish. Those three months remind me of how Sylvia Plath describes her psych ward neighbours in *The Bell Jar*: 'it was as if we had been forced together by some overwhelming circumstance, like war or plague, and shared a world of our own'.

My two pillars of support were Rubes and Vince, a cheeky ex-scaffolder who had the best arsenal of insults from years spent on building sites and a hard exterior, but turned out to be one of the sweetest people I know. He would whizz around the ward in his power chair and come to my bay to gossip most nights. There was a small kitchen where patients could practise carrying cups of tea and making food in occupational therapy sessions. The first meals Vince and I cooked in that kitchen after our injuries we shared with each other.

I was in a bad way one night, back on the ward after my first Christmas at home. A precious, brief taste of freedom. Hacer flew over to visit me while I was on home leave. She came into the kitchen, while I sat on the armchair in the corner, and I suddenly felt so small, so fragile. We cried together. She looked small too. We talked around the table and for some reason mimosas were mentioned. She had never heard of one and loved the idea of it. She has the ability to make anything magical, everything an event. She made me a mimosa every morning for the five days that I was home.

I had dreaded returning to hospital, but at the same time being home gave me a glimpse of the difficulties that were to come, a reminder that I was far from over the worst of this.

A deep sadness would come over me in those bleak winter days, a sadness that I did not know what to do with, that I could barely contain.

Dinner at Stanmore was always served inordinately early, and so I was in bed by seven, where I lay staring at the ceiling tiles, listening to one of the only five songs I could tolerate. Trying to sleep so I wouldn't have to think until I was woken up at six for breakfast.

Rubes wheeled into my bay and berated me for being in bed so early. I shrugged: what else was I supposed to do?

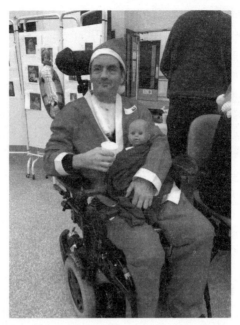

Vince in his Santa suit at the ward Christmas party.

He had come to show me the birthday cake his friends had dropped off for him. He always had a steady stream of visitors: university friends, family members, even his barber came to cut his hair. I found it too hard having people outside my immediate family here, letting them into this new, stark world. No one else needed to be witness to this.

The cake was clearly designed for a six-year-old girl; a large white fondant square decorated with pink icing flowers, and a plastic silver crown with pink jewels perched on top.

He put the crown on my head and dragged me out of bed. We fetched plastic knives and paper towels from the break room and began at the front of the spinal cord injury unit, delivering slices of cake to every bay of four patients.

The first bay was filled with mostly grumpy men. There was an older man whose spinal injury had happened years ago but came in with a pressure sore from a plane seatbelt. This gave me intense paranoia for years every time I flew.

Gerry the eccentric was also in this bay. He had tried on multiple occasions to convince me telepathy was real.

Then there was Will, who had fallen out of his wheelchair twice in the last week. Rubes and I were teaching him how to balance on his back wheels.

Finally we went to the women in the back bay. Edith, who I will much later be reminded of whenever I am faced with any older patient on a ward who won't stop talking about their toilet habits. Rachel, whose special subjects included the royal family, the cheek of Meghan Markle, and steak recipes.

Yvette was also here, and I could see that she had made peace with Edith over their warring around Yvette's radio volume. The conflict had lasted days, with Edith at one stage protesting by taking two white plastic cups that we usually drank our Movicol out of – a sickly-sweet laxative – and placing them over her ears. She looked like she was trying to make contact with an alien. She kept putting them back on whenever a nurse walked past to draw attention but everyone just ignored her. I think Yvette had won that one. Edith looked as if she'd lost the plot.

They seemed to have bonded over their hatred of dry

chicken and their love of Jersey unsalted butter. I saw a beautiful friendship forming.

Going back to the break room we bumped into Vince. He hated being in bed so much that he was always the first up in the morning and last to bed in the evening. He gladly took a piece of cake even though he's diabetic; he would always say yes to anything sweet.

We were living in a microcosm, each of us dealing with a harsh reality of our own; but it was a safe, small bubble. While it was incredibly painful it was also contained, comforting at times.

Fran spent weeks trying to find me a suitable wheelchair. I was too narrow for the adult ones they had on hand, so she went across the road to the paediatric ward to pick one up for me. When I went to the gym to try it out, to my horror, it had light-up front wheels, its metal frame encased in a bright orange lacquer. I sat in it and didn't know whether to laugh or cry at the absurdity. I did both.

I can think now how sweet for a disabled child to have light-up wheels, like the flashing Heelys we'd wear when I was young. But in that that moment it was my enemy.

A well-meaning nurse reassured me that once I had some experience in the outside world, I would be so much better at pushing up hills. I was aghast at her assumption I would still be a wheelchair user.

I felt such waves of hatred towards the wheelchair, even though, when thought of as a tool, like a pair of glasses, it could be nothing more than neutral. It took me years to see it as my independence, my autonomy, my mobility.

I would eventually come to recognise catheters in the same way; rather than a medical procedure, I began accepting them as a new way of living. As the key to my existence. My entire life, my entire future, depends on them. It becomes terrifying if I think about it too much. Every conversation, every moment of joy, laughter, connection, sadness, anger, grief, learning, I owe to these plastic tubes.

But early on, I still viewed any form of aid with hostility. I was fitted for a custom shower chair while in hospital; a chair I could roll over the toilet in, and into the shower to minimise the amount of transferring I would have to do. I was disturbed and embarrassed by the hole in the middle of the seat. I was so concerned that my friends would see it when they went into the bathroom, that I chose not to have it fitted over the toilet. At the time I would rather something be less functional for me than admit my needs to others.

After weeks of practising transfers from my wheelchair to various surfaces I was signed off to be allowed to get back into bed independently.

The first time I tried it on my own, I remember Edith was chatting away to me about something inane. I still blame her for distracting me.

'Do you need any help, Grace?' she said as I tried to inch myself forward from my wheelchair.

No, I was determined to do this by myself. But my

legs spasmed and my arms buckled, unable to get enough purchase on the bed.

'Oh . . .' Edith said as she watched me sink to the ground, legs collapsed into one another, my feet bent outwards in an unnatural position. Awkward and ungainly.

'. . . Should I call someone?'

I said yes through gritted teeth.

I remember the nurse was exasperated and told me off for trying on my own. I was angry with myself, felt as though I was failing.

After we had our induction to the accessible gym next to the hospital, patients were allowed to go there by themselves. I was so excited to be going somewhere unsupervised. I took the lift downstairs and entered the small gym area, aiming for the wheelchair treadmill. Unaware of the small but steep lip up to it, my front wheels tipped up and I instinctively leant back, my wheels spinning. I landed on the floor, hitting the back of my head. Unable to get back up, faces and hands appeared all around me. How many times I would fall and need to be lifted back on to bed, back on to my wheelchair. I was so deeply ashamed.

I'm alive, I'm alive, I'm alive, I would say to myself, for comfort.

Yet my mind went to wild places, too. Should my legs just be cut off? This is such an alarming thought process to me now; if part of a body is not useful, should it be removed? What is the point in it, if it doesn't function right?

Among the gifts of blankets, grapes, and Audible subscriptions I received from friends and family, I received a pair of beautiful cashmere socks. It made me so angry then: what was the use of them when I couldn't properly feel the socks on my feet any more? But did my poor feet not deserve cashmere if they could no longer feel it?

The much larger question I was dealing with, but could not articulate at that point, was this: what is the point in *me* if I don't function right?

There were moments when I felt such hatred towards my new state of being. I was faulty. I was the problem. I needed to be fixed. Some bone and nerves had realigned inside me to be inherently *wrong*. This was my harsh internal dialogue.

No wonder I felt this way. This is, after all, what the world tells us every day, in so many ways.

One fellow patient at Stanmore could walk but had little use of his hands. I was so envious of him early on, watching him wander around the break room. I was more interested in *looking* less disabled than having more function that would help me do the job I desired most. Minimising the visibility of my disability was paramount.

I was wrestling with such deep stigma, and ingrained aversion to disability. Looking back, I realise that newly injured people can be the most intensely ableist. There was a self-hatred that bubbled to the surface now that we found ourselves in this group of people we were likely to ignore before this.

It makes me wonder now how much of what I was experiencing was real grief, and how much of it was stigma rearing its head. A stigma I was suddenly forced to confront. I was experiencing a reckoning.

What had I thought of disabled people before my injury? What had I truly thought about our quality of life? Our value and worth?

Prognosis

Prognosis: from Greek *prognōsis*, from *pro-* 'before' + *gignōskein* 'to know'

What would become of me? I was beginning to wonder, waiting for my prognosis. Others knew, long before I would.

During my inpatient stay I had already experienced healthcare professionals projecting futures on to me: telling me how my skin would change, how I would need elbow replacements later in life now that I relied on my arms so much more, the drugs I would need, the pain I would experience. They gave me a glimpse into how I would be spoken to, treated.

But I was about to hear the prediction that mattered the most to me.

Six weeks into my stay at Stanmore, I had my official prognosis and diagnosis meeting. They had told me this meeting would happen at some point, after they had assessed my scans and looked at the progress I had made in physiotherapy, to discuss what my future mobility might be.

It felt like my judgement day.

In the few weeks prior, I had noticed that my feet could feel again. Not the same as before, but like a million pins and needles. Like electricity.

Every day I would get people to test them. I closed my eyes, and my parents or Nathan would touch me somewhere on my foot, and I would guess which foot and which part. It felt very important to me, for it to be true, to get it right. It felt like a promising start. Every time I worried that I would make a mistake, and it would turn out that I was just imagining it, my brain playing tricks on me.

I had vivid dreams about my legs, about walking again.

On the day of the meeting, we filed into Dr Wood's tiny windowless office.

She pulls out the plastic model of the spine she so often likes to use. She counts down the vertebrae from the top of the neck until she got to mine, C1, 2, 3, 4, 5, 6, T1, 2, 3, 4 – BINGO! That's where I was hit.

Then she points to the MRI of my spine on her computer screen. I was never very good at analysing scans as a student, but even I can see something is very wrong here. In a blur of white and grey and black, I see my long, pale grey spinal cord snaking down my back. Except halfway down it is disrupted, almost broken in two.

'We can't tell for sure what's going to happen, and there's always a chance that things will change any time; it's an incomplete injury, but on the more severe end of incomplete.'

The word 'severe' stings.

'The sooner things start changing, the better recovery is. It would be good to see things changing over the next few weeks, therefore.' It doesn't look hopeful, is what she's saying.

'How are you feeling, Grace?' she asks. Everyone's looking at me now.

'Okay,' I say. I'm not really sure what she wants me to say.

Dr Wood almost chuckles. 'Understatement of the century.'

I need to get out of this room as soon as possible.

We leave her office and I buckle in the corridor, folding over on to my legs. People are walking past so Nathan wheels me out into the car park.

There is a deep ache that runs from the pit of me through my lungs, out into a howl. I sob until there is no sound left, I cry until I am all dried up. I heave until all air is gone and I am gasping, choking on my own lungs. The heavens open – a pathetic fallacy of my pathetic situation.

Dr Wood joins us outside. She perches on the damp bench opposite me and explains it's not safe for me to go home yet. I hadn't trialled my outdoor visit yet.

I plead with her; I don't think I can face the bay after this. I desperately need to be anywhere but here.

I knew my diagnosis, but the prognosis, the permanence, had not hit until now when I was faced with that black and white image. My seemingly impenetrable bubble of denial had been burst. I imagine Dr Wood popping it with her painted fingernail. I had reached the end of a road that I thought would stretch on, and eventually lead me back to my old self.

This prognosis was a shock to me; I had tried so hard to progress during my hospital stay. While wheelchair skills classes felt like a chore, I had thrown myself into physiotherapy; practising standing up in wooden frames, rolling over on plinths, transferring to different surfaces, attaching patches to stimulate the muscles in my legs.

Every so often we would be tested to see if anything had changed.

'Tell me when you can feel this,' the physio would ask, placing one of his array of tools on my skin, first above the level of my injury. Easy. He would go down from my neck on to my chest until suddenly there was an absence. I'd close my eyes and will myself. Where was he touching me? I think I feel it – but do I know that because he's supposed to be touching me, or do I know that because I feel it? And where? The concentration would make my head pound.

It was an exam that I was bound to fail. He would hold my legs and ask me to push and pull against his hands. Nothing. Just silence, stillness.

I was so terrified of the prospect of 'no improvement' that when a nurse mistook my injury for *complete*, I was inconsolable. As if by design, I had become obsessed with these categories. I just had to progress to the next level.

My physio noticed one day that my lower back muscle 'flickered' when I concentrated hard enough. I reported this excitedly to Dr Wood, who brushed it off; it was insignificant. Maybe she was protecting me from a false hope, but her apathy was crushing.

I spent hours in bed at night willing just one toe to move. Scrunching up my eyes in concentration. Did it just twitch? Was I imagining it? Only to shine my phone torch under the blanket and see it still, as always.

As time went on, there was no improvement. My patchiness stayed the same and the flickers did not ignite into a full-blown flame.

Stanmore, through no fault of the staff, cultivated an atmosphere of competitiveness between patients, and because I was young, the assumption among others was that I *would* regain movement in my legs.

Everyone around me appeared to be making more progress than me. I felt as though something was irrevocably wrong inside.

Edith had started standing and taking steps on the parallel bars and would ask me nearly every day about my progress, eager to compare. The new patient diagonally opposite me would stop to tell me and my family in detail about all her movements in physiotherapy, and I would have to politely smile and say: well done!

I'm sure I was asked at least once a day by someone older than me, 'Are you walking yet?' as they made their way to the gym. Not yet, I'd say and smile. Not yet.

I made a folder on my laptop called '*Plan to hit this bitch*', with various links to articles, blogs, videos I'd found online of new exercises, new therapies to try. I wanted it to sound determined, to motivate me. I imagined triumphantly walking out of hospital, somehow victorious, as if this was something to defeat.

Of course I felt this way. Questions I would get about my 'recovery', from strangers to friends, often started with:

'Is there anything that can be done?'

'Are you getting better?'

'It's not permanent I hope?'

Five years later, I'm still asked these questions often. The implication is: 'Are you *always* going to be the way that you are?'

Because *this* was clearly not enough for people: my current being was insufficient. It was as if I was in a state of perpetual loading.

What was important was my physical recovery. To get back on my feet. Never mind what was going on inside my head – walking was the end goal. It was insidious, it was everywhere I turned.

A volunteer for one of the spinal charities, also a wheelchair user, would ask me every time she visited, 'Are you walking yet, Grace? No? Why not?'

I was too frightened, in those early days, to look at any scientific studies and risk hearing a prognosis I was not ready for. But there was more than enough on the internet to get started with.

I would discover that there is an entire industry for spinal cord injury 'cures', as some would describe: alternative movement therapies, suspicious supplements, prayers, people with questionable accreditations claiming they have a gift from God, charging a neat £250 an hour.

Even when I wasn't looking, Twitter messages from strangers filled my inbox, telling me if I meditated every day for a month I would wake up born again, renewed, damage undone. I would get comments about bizarre treatments that had apparently huge success, usually followed by a confusing anecdote about someone's great-aunt.

I am still regularly sent articles about an implant put into a rat's broken spine, allowing them to clamber around again with their little rat paws.

I AM NOT A RAT! I want to scream.

It is as though I am a lame animal, waiting for a cure or waiting to be put down. My cousin's sausage dog had a spinal cord injury quite soon after mine and had to be euthanised. It made me shiver.

I don't know what people want me to do with this information. Should I be thinking, *oh YES!* Thank God; now I'll just wait for them to do the simple transition from rat to human medicine and I will finally be freed from this purgatory.

It is so deeply ingrained in our society to equate disability with weakness, therefore using a wheelchair or any other mobility aid is an innate failing.

This narrative affects everyone. I see elderly people who are struggling to walk look at me with pity while I zoom past them. A friend told me about an old man who came up to her as she was handcycling, to say just how sorry he felt that she was in a wheelchair, as he slowly hobbled back across the street, unsteady. We laughed at the irony; how much his mobility could be improved with some assistance.

In my time at Stanmore, at first I thought I just needed to try harder. I wondered why a wheelchair user I knew who could cross his legs didn't keep trying, keep pushing to get more movement. That was what I had been told to do all my life: work hard, study hard, keep climbing up that wall.

The notion that some people don't want to be 'fixed', that they don't see anything that needs to be fixed in the first place, was unimaginable, incomprehensible to me.

Soon after that fated conversation in Dr Wood's office, in January, I had my case conference, a meeting with my team of physiotherapists, doctors, nurses, my occupational therapist, and case worker. Apart from Fran, it felt as though everyone had about as much empathy for me as for a cardboard box. It was after lunch, and my registrar looked like he could barely keep his eyes open.

I scanned around the room at these eight people looking at me. They were so far removed from what was happening to me inside. I tried to remind myself that for them, this was just another normal day at work; they will go home after this, they will make dinner, they will see their friends.

Dr Wood told me I was ready to go home, and there was nothing more they could help me with now. That I had run out of goals to achieve. I had reached the ceiling of progress here. I didn't feel ready at all. I thought there was more for me.

I was discharged two weeks later, on the 16th of January 2019.

Despite these meetings with professionals and finding little improvement in my physiotherapy sessions as a patient, I was determined to keep trying, to keep pushing for what I thought of then as a 'fix', once I was out of hospital.

We found a neuro-rehab centre on the outskirts of London, and my dad and I would make the four-hour round commute every week, where I would sit and will my legs to awaken, trying to telepathically communicate with them, as if I was trying to move an object on a table.

There is a video of me from March 2019, two months after leaving hospital, sitting on the kitchen counter, my legs dangling over the edge. I have pink streaks in my hair because I had just spent too much money and time at the hairdresser, desperate for change, desperately searching to find some kind of new identity for a self I didn't recognise. Perhaps I thought if I could change enough physically, I would come to find myself again.

I was grinning as I showed Nathan that if I pinched and tapped my thigh just above my knee and concentrated hard, my calf kicked forward. The kicks were small at first, and then there was one big swing out. It was an awkward, jerking movement, but a movement nonetheless.

I had made the discovery in my physio session earlier that day, and it felt like the start of something. It was *progress*. If I could do this, then what was next for me? I look young, naive, in that video.

Then I learned to stand, finally, by hauling myself up using a bar. My trainer would stop my knees from buckling and then they would lock for a few seconds in place, and I could hover my hands off the bar.

We took a photo and the picture looked good.

I looked triumphant, but I didn't feel strong inside. It

didn't feel right: I felt unsteady, immobile. It didn't feel the same as before my injury. This was all just for show.

I continued to try and move my legs further than the small kicks, but I couldn't connect with them. I considered making a movement with my lower body, but the message dissipated along the way, losing all meaning by the time it reached my legs. We weren't speaking the same language any more. The more I think, the more my leg buzzes; some sort of signal is getting down there, but it isn't the right one.

Desperate, I began looking into artificial ways I could appear to walk again. Calipers are metal splints that clip around your legs from your ankles to your hips, straightening the joints so you are able to swing your hips side to side, moving one leg like a pendulum inch by inch. Using calipers can be good for your bone density by weight-bearing, but otherwise, I didn't understand the appeal. Propped up by metal, I felt like a rag doll. I was so much less mobile, so much less independent, strapped to unyielding props.

But if I was eye to eye with people, perhaps I'd be treated like my pre-injury self. Was that the main motive?

Today, I see calipers as existing clearly for other people's benefit. Being held upright shows a superficial kind of improvement. It shows progress. To become like *everyone else* again. If I look the way I did before, it makes it easier for people to ignore that I'm disabled, and the inaccessibility of the world, the cynic in me thinks. It's a way to reverse the discomfort they feel at my situation. I will look 'better' to other people.

But who was I fixing myself for? And did I feel fixed in myself?

It took some time for the change in my own mindset to come, but when it did, there was no going back. I was sitting in the car with my dad one day, on our way to physio, when I heard myself speak the words out loud.

'I feel like everything I'm doing with my life now is for others.'

I was living life on someone else's terms, and it felt hollow. It took those eight months to dawn on me that, no matter what I did, this injury was permanent. No matter if I could stand again, or move my legs, there was no reversing the impact of an average-weight man landing directly on my spine from a great height.

There would be no way to change how I physically felt. My legs would always buzz with a numb electricity, I would most likely always rely on plastic straws to pee, nerve pain would be an unfortunate constant in my life.

Whether I *looked* disabled or not, the mountain of problems that come with a spinal cord injury that are not visible would still be there. There was no way to stitch up crushed nerves, to reconnect spindles, to fuse, weld – God, no amount of analogies I could use would reverse that day.

I had to stop forcing myself down the path that I had imagined for myself before my injury. That path had ruptured at my feet. If I didn't choose to change direction, I was going to fall away with it.

People can dedicate their life to the endeavour of progress, of walking again. They are applauded for this, for their motivation, for their strength. We lead different lives, and I don't judge such decisions, but it was not what I wanted.

I so envied people with spinal cord injuries who were able to walk, often termed 'Walkers', which makes them sounds like they belong in a zombie movie.

I began to realise that those that I knew in this category didn't seem necessarily happier than their seated friends. They had to grapple with the equally difficult task of living with an invisible disability, as people would imagine them 'cured' now that they were standing. It was assumed they needed no accommodations, no support – because physically they looked 'normal'.

I made the decision not to hold out for an abstract cure, or for my legs to wake up. No. Life was for living now. That meant embracing this wheelchair as a tool, a tool of mobility, of independence, not as a marker of failure. It meant accepting all of myself, rather than trying to fit into my old ideas of perfectionism and striving. Seeking a new definition of recovery; one that is not objective, linear or wholly physical. One that can be a small smile, a joke, a laugh, a deep breath out. When things no longer feel so frightening. The beginnings of acceptance. Anchored once more to a sense of self.

I began to see that recovery is coming back to yourself again.

I began to feel that some of that was happening to me.

Early on it was easy for me to imagine that if only I could stand up, then I would be happy again. Then, if only I could move my legs more, I would be happy; then if I only I could – and on and on and on.

But this is a hopeless way to be, to focus on what you lack in life, constantly chasing something unquenchable, always out of reach.

I've started to reframe desire. What makes me feel good now? What serves me well? What makes me feel alive? What is progress, for me? What does recovery look like within these parameters?

Juan made me consider this early on. Soon after I was discharged, he came to visit me. He could see how flat I was, how lost. He made me sign up to the local gym, and twice a week we wheeled there together. He didn't try to help me; as hard as it was he wanted me to push my wheelchair the whole way. We did the route again and again until I figured out the smoothest way to go. He would get me a coffee from the café and then we'd go into the gym.

We'd laugh about the music and the motivational quotes in the windowless room where the weights are kept; it is very different from the light and airy climbing gym where we had spent years together as I was growing up.

We'd practise wheeling back and forth as fast as I could. We'd practise picking things up from the floor, by holding on to one wheel and leaning down to grab a weighted ball, slowly rolling it up the side of the wheel until it is on my lap. These are techniques I still use every day. This was real progress for me.

Juan didn't ask me if I was getting better. He took me as I was, each day.

*

I had been home a few months before I returned to the Stanmore for a repeat MRI scan, to ensure my spine and spinal cord looked stable, which they were. I remember the radiographer asking me about the bruise on my toe. It looked quite different to when I woke up with it the morning after my injury.

New growth was starting to show – I saw new nail growing upwards, sprouting through. At the same time, the muscles around my spine grew back over the surgical metal rods, like tendrils around park railings.

I had spent hours in my hospital bed, willing my toes to move, and that red and purple and brown bruise on my big toe would stare back at me, unchanging. Now it was inching up my nail, soon it would not be there at all. I was recovering in some ways I did not expect, and not in others.

It felt strange, to start to feel content in a state I had been told was not enough. It was difficult for others to understand this. To accept my acceptance. I felt like they didn't believe me when I would say I was happy, as if I had to convince them otherwise, give them examples of how well I was now doing.

I was lucky. I had the space and support to look at a cure in a different way; a loving and devoted partner and family, the ability to get suitable, well-fitted and designed mobility equipment, financial help, housing security. I did not have to rely on old-fashioned ideals of 'wellness'. I could make my own normal.

I was not following the path of what I might once have seen as 'real' recovery. In films, a three-minute montage of a hero clutching parallel bars, inching their way across them. Taking their first steps, for the second time. The viral local news story of a person walking again against all odds. It is a story of overcoming, of resilience, of physicality, of perseverance.

On social media we crave a quick fix: plastic surgery, before and after weight loss pictures, learning to walk again. It is satisfying seeing things 'righted', to align with society's ideals once more.

All is right with the world again.

I saw another common theme in these recovery stories on social media – the trope of 'proving doctors wrong'. The headline usually reads something like: Doctors told me I would never walk again/I would never dance again/I would never smile again/I would never whatever again, followed by a triumphant video of them defiantly doing that exact thing they were told they would NEVER do. I have exceeded all expectations and look at me now! I am better!

I am sure doctors can often underestimate a person's willpower or extent of recovery, but when I read these, I imagine a doctor shaking their fist at someone: 'Oh, I told you never to dance again!'

No one told me that I would never walk again, but my consultant strongly suggested it was unlikely, and as much as I hated her approach, she was right. Perhaps I am at exactly the physical level doctors predicted, and that's okay. This is not something I need to overcome; this is not a hurdle set in front of me.

It is not a barrier to me. It means a different way of life, maybe, but it's not a barrier.

I realised that I *would* be cured, but not in the way I once envisaged.

My cure came in the form of community, of anger, of activism.

Outside

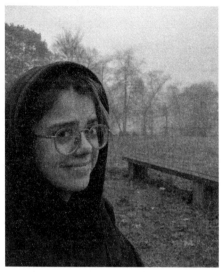

Nathan sneaked me outside of Stanmore for the first time,
only to find fields. My facial expression says it all.

Sooner than I perhaps felt ready for I was discharged,
and a new life began.

I went through periods of normality, getting bothered
by everyday things that everyone gets bothered by; a
window back into life before, when little things would
be irritating.

Often – almost daily – I went through periods of low.
Such low that I could barely breathe in the agony of it
all. It felt like there was a gaping hole where my life used

to be. Then I would feel joy I don't know if I've ever felt before, joy I don't know whether people who haven't had such a significant experience could feel.

I was grateful to be alive before, sure, but not in this way. The winter sun reflected on the trees in orange, red and green. The fairy lights cascading down a pub window. The dappled pattern of light reflecting on the bottom of a pool. The sunlight from a window through a white sheet hung up to dry. The feeling after a hot shower when I turn off the water and I am warm and clean. It was all so overwhelming.

These moments are the most beautiful I've ever experienced. Lights shine harder now, colours are more piercing. The world is so beautiful that I can't believe I get to witness it.

It was intense, and loud. Like I had been living in a dark, tasteless place for many months and suddenly switched into technicolour.

I wanted to be so grateful for life, but I also felt that I no longer had a place in it. How could I retain these small moments of joy when faced with such pain, such difficulty?

Whereas I was so at ease in the world before, so ready to enter any room, now I have been dropped into deep water and I cannot swim.

As soon as that man's head met my back, I joined a different group in society. The world – so open to me before as a privileged, young white woman – now felt hostile. I was disabled, but only beginning to grasp what that meant.

*

I had never noticed how uneven the paving stones were on the street of my parents' house. How many steps there were up to the front door. How the wobbly wooden floorboards now creaked under my wheels.

How full of challenges my home was now. I couldn't even shower there. The doctors had suggested I stay in a hotel if my parents' house wasn't adapted for me yet, 'to treat it as a holiday', when it felt the furthest thing from that.

To my dismay I realised how many places I was barred from entering. Whether because there were steps and no lift, a broken lift, a lift too small to fit a wheelchair, no disabled toilet, an invariably *broken* disabled toilet, narrow corridors, awkward seating: it all served as a constant reminder that I was no longer designed for this world. It was a jarring transition.

I no longer looked like anyone else I knew and found that in many places my presence was not expected, or desired.

I was on the other side of the glass looking in, often literally.

The change in my bodily state was difficult for friends to navigate and led to some avoiding seeing me at all. Was I too complicated for them now? Did I make them too sad? It made me wonder.

Invitations now came with certain conditions. I could come but I would have to be picked up and carried somewhere; I could come but I wouldn't be able to use the bathroom; I could come to the first part, but not the second. Failing all of this, I would not be invited at all.

To my dismay, a close friend early on asked if he

should tell me when he and our group of friends were doing something that I would not be able to do. I had not realised there were so many things they had decided I couldn't do.

I don't blame them for these early interactions. We were all trying, all learning to navigate new territory, but it felt as though my life had suddenly become smaller, and with that the people around me had shrunk their view of me, of my abilities. I was being counted out before I even had a chance to try. Often, I felt as though my presence hadn't been considered when people were making plans, but not only that – I felt that it wasn't desired. Oh, what a horrible feeling. It became so normalised to be excluded that I felt I had to be grateful whenever I was included. Pleasantly surprised. The bar was suddenly very low, and I got used to it.

Pub managers and venue owners would often tell me that they didn't get many disabled people at their establishment, to excuse why they didn't know basic information about their facilities. I would think: No shit, Sherlock, of course you don't, I can't make it in the door!

And so the cycle of inaccessibility, exclusion and poor design continues.

I began to imagine a video game-style red hue crashing down over every place I could no longer access. My whole field of vision became tinged with red.

I was learning that even when I am able to enter a play, concert, even a restaurant, many times I'm ushered in the 'accessible' way, usually down an alley, through a back door, past store cupboards, kitchens, staff rooms. Hidden from view, with the bins.

I fight to get in lifts, I manoeuvre through dark corridors. I am constantly reminded I am an extra, an afterthought.

I found that there were many ways I was actively excluded, and many ways this was done passively. When I am not able to physically enter through the door, that's a clear message. But even where there may be a lift, and an accessible toilet, there might be some less obvious ways I'd be left out. For instance, one education centre in medical school was accessible, but had only bar-style stools and high tables in the break rooms. I had to eat my lunch at eye level with people's knees. A hostile design, for those who don't fit a certain mould. It made me wonder, does it matter if I can enter the room, if I then can't reach a seat at the table?

I was learning that, as disabled people, we have designated places to occupy, often sidelined and separate. That there were set assumptions on who we might want to bring or hang out with – just one personal assistant. God forbid I would want to go out with multiple friends.

Thanks to Stanmore, I had just about got to grips with using catheters and built up a routine, and now wanted to know how I was to tackle these procedures in a bathroom that was not my own. This had been much less of a focus during my rehab, which made me suspect that they did not expect me to have much of a social life.

I was anxious. The hospital had been such a contained space; how would I fare in public? How would I manage in the pub, in a restaurant, out on a picnic?

Although I had just about learned to do these things independently at home, my strict schedule suddenly didn't fit with the life I wanted to lead, if I ever planned on leaving the house for more than four hours at a time.

I left rehab sort of knowing how to do it all in *theory*, but with no confidence outside of the ward. I have never felt more alone than on those first times I tried to catheterise in a toilet far from home, without help. It was only when I was faced with life outside of the hospital that I realised how limiting this could be, how difficult. This huge part of my life that was never talked about, that people didn't know about, let alone understand.

I was almost entirely reliant on happening to find infrastructure that considered me and bodies like mine, and I was often realising that, for the most part, the world did not. I only truly realised the importance of public bathrooms when I was suddenly denied them.

How many toilets have I had to use with the door open as I don't fit, guarded by friends? What gymnastics have I had to do in an attempt to get from my wheelchair seat to an awkwardly placed toilet? How many 'accessible' bathrooms have I come across that are most often locked, broken or have been co-opted as a storage closet, forcing me to manoeuvre around furniture, signs, cleaning products, only to sit on oddly shaped toilet seats that make me feel as though my hip is about to dislocate.

Access to clean, safe bathrooms is a human right. In the UK, legally every establishment over a certain size should have a disabled bathroom but, in reality, this is so often not the case. And 'minimum statutory guidelines' often fall short of what we actually need. As soon as I do not have access to a bathroom, I am excluded. This is such a barrier to engaging in society, in life – as well as a source of pain, a feeling of worthlessness.

Disabled toilets are also where some of my most awkward encounters with strangers tend to happen. People with invisible disabilities are well within their right to use these bathrooms, of course, and might have a harder time navigating this if they do not look like they require it. But this is clearly not what's going on, however, when I find myself waiting and waiting outside an accessible bathroom, and a group of friends come out having used it as a changing room, and they see me, and begin to apologise, look at each other sheepishly, giggling.

I remember a friend at university when we were in second year recounting how he walked out of a disabled toilet to find someone *actually* disabled waiting outside, and how embarrassed he was. I remember laughing. I am sure I have been the disabled stranger in the punchline of many stories by now.

It is comical to me at times, how people will react when they come out of the toilet and see me; the dance we must do, the apologies, the sidestepping, the look of surprise, the gasps.

I ignore it most of the time. I don't want a fuss, I don't even care if they've used it; I just don't want this uncomfortable meeting. But if you're so embarrassed to be faced with me now, why did you use it in the first place? I want to ask.

Disabled toilets have been the setting of more disturbing encounters too. One in particular stands out.

I had just finished seeing friends for a drink. Everyone

was leaving, so I went back into the pub on my own. I was desperate to pee after a pint of Guinness, and relieved to find they had an accessible toilet.

I go in, but as soon as I transfer on to the toilet I hear the handle rattle. I hate this sound. It is passive-aggressive, verging on plain aggressive. I admit I have done it before, when you're desperate and you feel as though you need to remind the person inside that someone is waiting. This particular rattle is angry already. I say, 'Sorry! Occupied!' Like I normally do.

I am trying not to panic in these situations any more, trying to remind myself I deserve to be able to pee just like everyone else. I try not to rush, take a deep breath. Then I hear a knock at the door.

'HOWAY!'

A strong Geordie accent comes from the other side. I am not frightened yet, just a little confused.

BANG BANG BANG

'HOWAY MAN!'

Again, it is louder. She sounds exasperated as if she has been waiting half an hour when I have been in the bathroom all but two minutes. I have a somewhat delicious feeling at the thought of the look on her face when she sees me.

I tell myself to take a deep breath – you will get out of this situation. But I feel trapped in this moment when I hear it again:

BANG BANG BANG

It's angrier now and sounds as if she is banging on the door with both fists.

'HOWWAYYY MAN!!'

I am shouting back now that I'll just be a minute. I can hear her grumbling and then she shouts:

'HAVE YOU GOT A FUCKING DISABILITY OR WHAT?'

'Yes, I'm a wheelchair user!' I shout back, thinking, hoping this will surely put a stop to this. She will be subdued.

'I don't believe you . . . the fuck you do.'

She is sneering at me. I cannot believe the anger, the vitriol, of this voice on the other side of the door.

To my horror, now I hear a man's voice speak. He is telling the woman how she can open a locked door. As if it is a fun trick he has learned, he describes how to press your nail into the screw of the lock, and twist.

Before I can protest, I can hear the door beginning to click. I am shouting at this point, pleading, it becomes a blur. I am completely incapacitated, and I can hardly leap up to stop her from doing this.

I am still on the toilet, in my most vulnerable position. The door opens, but only slightly, not enough for me to see her, but enough for her to see me. It is obvious she has seen my wheelchair because the door closes again quickly. It is still unlocked, slightly ajar.

I am stunned. I pull on my trousers, shaking. I want to hurry to catch her, to shout, to question. I wheel out, slamming the unlocked door open, but there is no one in the corridor now.

I frantically look around the pub, see so many faces laughing, talking, many of my colleagues, unaware that I have just been violated by a stranger. As if it was a figment of my imagination. Horrible voices in my head.

I call Nathan in tears. He cycles from work immediately. I am torn whether to leave. I feel the opportunity to confront, to stand up for myself was taken away by the cowardice of whoever was behind that voice running away.

We stay outside the pub a little longer. I am becoming despondent, so we turn to leave when I hear the voice behind the door again, the same accent, the same gravelly tone, the same inflection.

I turn around, and ask her, was that you in the toilet just then?

She denies it but is too drunk to be able to lie convincingly. She avoids eye contact with me, looks down at the floor. She grabs her friend, and they begin to run up to the main road and vanish. I look for her.

My tears turn to laughter. She is hiding behind a lamp post.

We accost them in the street, Nathan pulls his phone out to film them. I hear myself shouting now: 'HOW DARE YOU?'

That sneering voice comes out again. 'WE ARE ACTUALLY CARERS,' she says, stumbling along the street. They bundle into a taxi and we leave too, laughing.

I now have a ridiculous video of me shouting at two middle-aged women drunk out of their minds, dropping their vapes.

I could have reported them, but this felt good enough. I could not tolerate victimising myself further. It's one of my worst fears realised: to be violated AND not believed.

Am I not even safe in the place designated for me?

After writing this I have a nightmare that it's happening

again, and it's enough to wake me up, heart pounding, shaking, trying to catch my breath.

Luckily this is far from a regular occurrence, and no one else since has invaded the bathroom to see if I *really* am disabled, but it illustrated to me the way that disabled people are continually intruded on. Violations of personal space, of personal information take many forms. We constantly need to prove ourselves, prove that we're not faking it. Our right to privacy is always in question.

It becomes demeaning to regularly have to ring ahead or go in and ask places if they have a toilet I can use, and then be faced with staff discussing whether they think I will fit, imagining me in their particular toilet cubicle. Normally people are overconfident about the accessibility of their space, and so once I have tried, I then have to explain to everyone I'm with why it doesn't work for me, that I will need to go elsewhere.

Everyone uses a bathroom in one way or another, but disabled people must announce it to the world, declare it loudly on arrival. We are not given any privacy.

I was filled with shame early on after my injury, I did not want to share my needs with others. I would spend hours in pain through a desperation to pee, pretending to friends that everything was fine while we stayed for an extra drink in inaccessible places.

The bathroom is a space where ableism occurs on every scale. It is a microcosm of society, an indicator of who we want to let in or leave out. They are the places where infrastructure, stigma and societal priorities collide. They can be used as a tool of oppression, of exclusion – or one of equity, a way to signal who is welcome. The agent of great change, of freedom, of inclusion.

Toilets were just the start. There were so many large and small shifts in my world, after discharge.

I found not only did my physical needs change how I could access spaces, the way I looked radically changed how people interacted with me once I got there.

Some people had a physical reaction to seeing me, looking visibly uncomfortable with my appearance, as if I was causing them pain.

Some people felt they must address it straight away, maybe making a joke about my speed, my driving skills.

'Must be hard on your fingers!!'

'No speeding!'

'Have you got a licence for that!'

'Don't run over my toes!'

I have had people stumble over their words so many times. People saying, 'let's walk this way', and then apologising for using the word *walk*, as if it would cause offence.

Strangers sometimes appeared averse to touching me, as if I am infectious, as if I will spread whatever has made me a wheelchair user to them, whether from awkwardness, or genuine anxiety. They would leap out of my way, apologise for being two metres away from me.

'I know, I know, it's okay, it's okay!'

'You're okay – you're all right!'

These things I would say on repeat, smiling while

they fluster. To begin with I felt like I had to comfort other people, for the difficulty they were having with the wheelchair.

I found that my private life was not so private. That there is a certain intrigue, that people want answers when it comes to disabled people, and feel like they deserve them. On the one hand, I would have loved for people to have an awareness and an understanding of what I needed, but at the same time I didn't want to satisfy their morbid curiosity. There is such a tension here.

There was a curiosity around my body now too. An eagerness to know about my bodily functions, in a way that is not motivated by a desire to help, that wouldn't lead to any productive action, it's just a desire to *know*.

It reminded me of the voyeurism people sometimes direct towards trans people having gender reassignment surgery, this obsession with another's genitals.

Suddenly it felt as though nothing was mine to keep.

I was beginning to understand that this curiosity is not born from the individual, that it has come from hundreds of years of society's somewhat grotesque fascination with disabled people. Until recently the only place to commonly see us was on charity television programmes; confessing our most intimate health diagnoses in exchange for public donations. Not so long before that we were a part of circus shows or locked in institutions. The curiosity with those who look, communicate and move differently is so ingrained, so normalised. We are an unnerving presence and we're expected to perform.

*

I was learning too that it didn't have to be this way.

I found to my relief that it *was* possible to have conversations around disability. Things go far better when curiosity is directed towards how I navigate the world, how I interact with the barriers I face, rather than digging into the supposed integral problems with *me*. I would much rather talk about the tread of my wheelchair tyres, how my motorised wheel attaches, how I can be supported, how I have progressed, what I've learned.

It is refreshing to talk not about what's supposedly 'wrong', but rather about my adaptations, my perspective, how we can remove barriers together. I don't want some apology for who I am, or my supposedly sad situation, or to satisfy a stranger's voyeurism.

When I get close to someone, sometimes I do want them to know my story, my past. I want them to know where I have been, where I will go. But as with any difficult period in anyone's life, it is not usually something to be shared right away. I want to build a relationship of trust, and it may come up naturally, or it may not. Disabled people deserve that choice too, that control.

While some people can be abrupt, tactless, it's just as common to find people struggling to say what they mean at all, frozen by a fear of offending or getting the words wrong, skirting around with vague language. 'Do you have trouble finding your way with . . . this?' they might say, gesturing vaguely at me up and down. Go on, SAY IT! As if they think that when they say the words 'wheelchair' or 'disabled' out loud, I will suddenly realise, I will be reminded of my own misfortune. I have heard so many euphemisms – I guess used to try and soften the blow. Person living with a disability (as if it is my pet), differently abled, less abled, persons of determination (yes, a real one), which to me all further stigmatise, further suggest I should be ashamed.

People have told me they don't see me as disabled, as if this is a compliment. But I need people to please see ALL of me. If you don't see me as disabled, then you are not looking at me properly, I want to say. You are missing a huge part of me by trying to ignore this.

I often wonder if disabled people were more visible across society, would this be the case? I have found that once I spend time with someone new, they become much more comfortable with me. Repeated exposure to seeing someone use a wheelchair means they get used to it, all anxiety evaporating.

I notice this even as a patient. When I see the same healthcare professional a few times, the dynamics change so quickly. I remember my first appointment with a particular nurse at my GP: she was so anxious, worried about how I would move around the clinic room, she was talking too much, getting flustered. The next time I saw her the difference was astounding.

When I was first injured, many friends couldn't help but treat me as fragile goods, unsure how my new body worked and interacted with the environment. The way my legs abruptly spasm, the way I sometimes have to hold myself up by my elbows, appears foreign at first.

But the more they began to understand my life, and saw the way I moved, the more comfortable they became. It didn't take long – a few conversations, people are quick learners. Today, I can immediately recognise when someone I meet has had this experience already or has disabled friends or family.

When I was first injured, I thought if I could be like the doctor on the television show *House* and walk with a golden cane, then maybe it would all be worth it; I'd be mysterious, interesting. It made Nathan cry on his cycle home, this naive hope. I had left the Royal London clinging on to the idea that this would all be reversed, a funny story to tell one day. The only remnant a cane. Did I fixate on that vision as it was the only representation I had seen? I didn't know any visibly disabled people, so what else could I go on?

This hope signified to me early on that there is an *acceptability* of certain disabilities, a hierarchy within the community. What is a palatable disability? Who is allowed to be represented in mainstream media?

In some ways I am hypervisible; I am the symbol of accessibility; I match the disabled toilet sign! I have to acknowledge that this means, as a manual wheelchair user, I can have an easier time in the public eye, and I am more likely to be represented than people who communicate differently. Who have facial differences, who have learning disabilities, who are power wheelchair users – let alone considering the intersectional challenges many people face. There are many layers of stigma people have to work against.

But there is a dearth in the representation of *all* of us.

It is no surprise, then, that we are treated with such bewilderment. When I enter a room or someone steps into the room I'm in, I have learned to expect a gasp, a look of surprise, even an exclamation in some circumstances. Nowadays, I'm very used to my state of being, so I find it bizarre. Am I really the first wheelchair user they have ever spoken to?

At this point, when I'm faced with a strange question or comment, I can be taken aback, simply because I have forgotten momentarily how I am perceived. As other wheelchair user friends have joked, we don't exactly go around Sainsbury's and think: 'Here I am, a wheelchair user!'; we just think, I need to get eggs, bread and milk.

It is the lack of information about the real lives of disabled people that leads to this lack of awareness, which in turn leads to these uncomfortable situations. Fundamentally, exclusion creates ignorance, ignorance creates fear, suspicion. Awkwardness.

It explains why I was so lost after my injury and confused about my new identity. I had no idea how disabled people really lived, or what life would be like, because I had not seen us anywhere.

PART 3:
Reformation

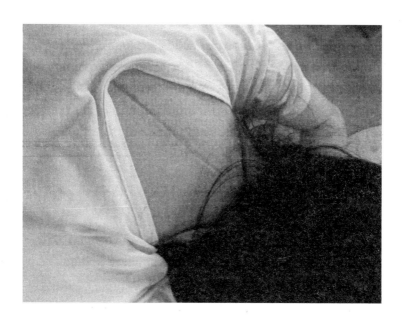

Caring

Nowadays when I see patients at work, or a family member in hospital, I can understand how they feel their stay is never going to end. I know what it is to feel that you're never going to get out of it, you can't imagine a way forward, can't see a new life ahead of you. You are in a black hole.

And then one day, suddenly, it is all a memory.

I had always wanted to be able to look after people, to put them at ease, to provide comfort. I come from a family of caregivers: doctors, nurses, physiotherapists, occupational therapists and social workers – enough to make up an entire multidisciplinary team.

I'd hear stories of my mother as a student taking people in; she was everyone's confidante when I was growing up. Our house was a place of refuge for so many passing through. I saw how giving she was, and how effortless she made it all seem. She was so busy but was always able to pick people up along the way. She had the gift of being able to give people unquestioning, unconditional support.

I wanted to emulate her; spending hours in the garden patching up a butterfly's wings, building a training area for it to learn to fly again. Meticulously gluing together a mosaic prosthetic shell for a broken snail. Even as a very small child, taking care of people gave me purpose and made me feel in control, when my brain so often didn't.

When I was fourteen, a girl in my class died by suicide, one early morning, alone in her garden. It was 2011 and Facebook was the centre of every fourteen-year-old's world, and so I heard the news the way no death should ever be found out, when everyone began to post heart emojis on their statuses after school.

One of my best friends came to stay that night. She was in foster care at the time and had been closer to the friend who had died. We slept in bed with my mum, and I remember her crying, my mum comforting her. I must not cry out, I thought to myself, I am not the one in the most grief. Like so many of us do, I put other people's pain above my own.

She had a Jewish funeral in North London. The rabbi called her a flower plucked from earth. We walked from the synagogue to her grave, sobbing. There was nothing good to come of this, no lessons, no celebration of life, only sorrow.

It was the first glitch in a reality that had felt so secure. A chasm had opened up before my feet where I thought was solid ground. People my age weren't supposed to die.

How could this have happened? Was there something I could have done? I vowed to never let it happen again, as if it had ever been something I could control. I would not fail again. I must know better next time.

If only I had known how she was feeling, if only I'd had the tools to help her. I vastly overstated my abilities to alter the course of events. These feelings of fear, inadequacy and sense of guilt carried on into my early twenties. Friends would have mental health crises and I would take the burden on myself. I thought if I just stayed with people at all times, they couldn't hurt themselves. I felt guilty all the time, about letting people down, about disappointing them.

I had such a clear picture in my head of the role of the doctor as someone in control, someone who could help people, and this was the role I wanted to play in life. I had always wanted to be a fixer and early on was determined on applying to medical school to do this.

After my injury, I wondered how on earth would this be possible, how I could still be capable in this new body, which felt so unyielding, so beyond my control. I couldn't imagine looking after others when I barely knew how to look after myself.

The head of the medical school and head of year four and five students had visited me in the very early days of my injury, when I was still in the high-dependency unit. They said I could absolutely continue in medicine and that they would support me with this. I appreciated their resolve, but at the same time I thought: how could they possibly know? Two able-bodied men being so sure did not fill me with confidence. I had never seen a visibly disabled healthcare worker before.

*

I had been called a 'forever patient' early on in my hospital stay. It was supposed to be reassuring; my spinal unit would always be there for support and advice even after my discharge, but the term filled me with dread. Who wants to be a *forever* patient? How can I be a doctor if I will always be a patient? To be both, concurrently, felt completely incongruous.

There was no middle way in my mind, as I began to grapple with a new identity that felt so at odds with the life I had imagined. I didn't know of anyone who was both, who straddled these two identities. On the contrary, to get through the gruelling university course there did not seem to be any space to be ill, or take time off, let alone be disabled.

To be a doctor was to be healthy. I felt far away from that, still attached to a bed by drains and tubes.

Later, when I was moved to Stanmore, some hope sparked in me. One of the psychologists who worked on the unit was a wheelchair user. I could not believe my eyes as she rolled around the ward, seeing patients. I desperately wanted to talk to her, to find common ground and see something of what I might become in her.

When I was discharged, I scoured the internet and found a doctor in Scotland who was also a wheelchair user. I reached out to her, and we spoke on the phone for two hours. She was funny and determined and filled me with comfort. That call with her shored up something within me. She could not give me an idea of every obstacle I would face, but she gave me a picture, a vision I could work towards. I knew it would be hard, but if someone else was doing it, I should be able to.

Knowing this meant everything.

I returned to medical school ten months after my spinal cord injury. I was eager to get back to medicine, but it seemed that medicine wasn't ready for me.

I remember my first time observing in theatre as a wheelchair user. I was so nervous; I had barely mastered getting dressed and undressed while sitting in my wheelchair, and now I had to rush to put on scrubs in front of the other medical student who I'd only met days before. I felt so self-conscious, fumbling in my attempt to pull the loose scrub trousers up to my waist, unable to reach both hands above my head to put the top on without folding on to my knees.

We were observing an orthopaedic theatre list – hip replacements, spinal surgeries, a lot of physical work – and the consultant surgeons lived up to the unfortunate stereotype: unfriendly, cold. They made it clear there was no role for me. At one stage one even joked about being close to paralysing a patient on a previous case.

They made me feel so small, so insignificant in that room. I left and cried in the changing room. I felt so alone. Who could I talk to about this? I was in a new year of students, and barely knew anyone.

Did you think you could fit in here? You do not belong, was the message I heard, loudly.

I soon found that fellow students and senior doctors didn't quite know what to do with me or how to talk to me now that I was seated. I felt like the special case; other students would be assigned tasks and then a senior doctor would lean towards me: 'we'll find something for you to do, Grace'.

My abilities were vastly underestimated, and often I didn't feel as though I got the opportunity to try anything out. It was already assumed it would be too difficult for me.

As a wheelchair user, doing all the practical, physical activities on the wards was hard to get accustomed to at first. Fitting in tiny handover rooms, battling with trying to open foot pedal bins, high shelves out of reach, but it was just as challenging getting to grips with the classes and the way we were taught, after all I had experienced. I felt I could relate much more to the patient pictured on the slide than the lecturer.

I was so nervous wheeling into the first lecture of fourth year, in a cohort I did not know, but assumed most knew what had happened to me. I wanted to be quiet, to blend in. This was difficult when the only accessible place in this lecture theatre, as is usually the case, is right at the front.

Soon after the lecture started, I dropped my pen. I froze, not completely comfortable with bending down yet terrified that I would struggle to do this simple task in front of everyone. The lecturer noticed my predicament, paused their talk to the hundred people in the room, asked if I need help picking it up. I shook my head, crimson, too terrified to draw attention to myself. I went without a pen.

The content of these lectures was hard to face at times. How many teaching sessions I sat in, feeling completely out of place, while my condition was talked about as the worst-case scenario. A disaster, to be avoided at all costs. The negativity and catastrophising around illness, disability and difference felt so stark, so personal now. I had skin in the game.

I listened while lecturers advised on preventing spinal cord injuries: don't miss it, don't leave it, treat quickly. Why is someone off their legs? That's not normal. Do you see a change in bowel and bladder movements? That's not normal. During these talks, I felt like everyone's eyes were boring into the back of my head, as one consultant hammered home the point that these symptoms are an emergency, and if left untreated the patient can become *fully paraplegic*.

It is important to be taught these topics, of course, but it is hard to be reminded that your life is the worst-case scenario. I wondered if the choices made around the way this is taught changes how these patients are treated, if they do have one of these 'catastrophic' diagnoses.

How can you not treat these patients in a certain way if you believe they are at the end of the road? It felt like this purely medical approach left no room for the possibilities and potential richness of a disabled life.

It also left no room for the priorities of a disabled person, which I was realising may be very different from those of an able-bodied one.

I know my priorities and needs now appeared foreign to some healthcare professionals; that I wanted vaccinations administered in my leg as I relied on my arms too much, that the length of time I'd have to sit or lie on a surface had to be minimal to avoid pressure sores, that being able to lift my hands above my head to tie my hair up was so important to me. Specific, functional things that related to my daily life were hard to understand if someone couldn't conceptualise me out of the clinic room.

It was obvious, by how awkward some of my fellow students were towards me, that these might be their first interactions with a visibly disabled person. They would undoubtedly meet many disabled people at work, more so than the general public, so this concerned me.

These lectures were a constant reminder that I was unlike the rest of my cohort. I don't think most other doctors have to think about their personal life, question their worth so intimately at work.

Every new placement I had as a student, staff would try their best to accommodate me, but the old-fashioned NHS buildings presented many challenges. You'd be lucky to find accessible staff toilets in most hospitals, but it's pretty much unheard of to find accessible locker rooms, or staff kitchens. These areas were never designed with a thought that someone like me would ever be working there.

I was constantly reminded that I was playing the wrong role.

Whenever I needed to get a taxi into the hospital for placement the driver would tell me that they hoped my appointment went well. I had (and still have) regular awkward encounters with colleagues who at first think I am a patient. Ignoring the lanyard, the stethoscope, the scrubs: the sight of a wheelchair eclipses all.

Back then, I felt so much pressure, so much weight on me, that I feared I would break.

I had written the words *I am not scared of anything any more* in my diary on the 8th of December, seven weeks after my spinal cord injury. One of the worst things my small head could imagine had happened, and although it felt disastrous, I was still waking up every day. Still eating breakfast, still joking with Vince and Rubes, still laughing at Will falling out of his wheelchair, still writing everything down. I was still *here*. As fragile as I felt, it also made me feel quietly invincible at first.

But I struggled to hold on to this feeling of fearlessness once I was out of hospital, out in the real world again. I was vulnerable to everything. I cried all the time, defenceless to the microaggression upon microaggression that were piling up. I felt like a blank canvas for others to impress their assumptions upon, to paint me in broad strokes. How could I protest? I didn't know if I had any part of me left to object, and besides many of the assumptions and prejudices were ones I so recently held myself.

Was this the way I would be treated now?

I still felt as though I had to be nice to everyone, grateful for everything, the pleasant and polite disabled girl, spoken over, spoken about, ignored. This need to absorb, diffuse and placate, think of other people's feelings first, is so deeply ingrained in women, in particular. I had always been so desperate to be good. But this approach to life wasn't going to cut it any longer, thrust into the public, no longer in the protective circle of friends and family in which I had been safely enclosed since being discharged.

By January 2020, it felt too heavy to carry any longer. I couldn't bear having any more arguments with myself in the shower, after the fact, saying everything I wished I could have said in response to the latest slight or patronising comment. There is no satisfaction in talking to a tiled wall. Something needed to change, or I would lose myself completely in the tidal waves of other people's projections.

I hadn't spoken to a professional since leaving Stanmore. I reached out to some therapists I found online. One tells me their office is inaccessible, so they instead suggest a colleague of theirs. I make an appointment with the therapist they recommend, not knowing much about her.

I waited anxiously for my session. I had not been to therapy since my second year of medical school when I was dealing with some debilitating anxiety. How could I explain to this stranger the recent overwhelming, complicated events of my life, where I am now, the challenging ideas I was dealing with? How would they be able to understand any of it? How could they possibly guide me through this total mess?

I had been to a trial session with a different therapist the previous week. She had appeared overwhelmed, a little lost by my summary of the strange recent events in my life. I had left feeling even more alone.

This time, my therapist emerged from her consulting room to call my name, and I realised that she was also disabled. I could barely contain my shock; my mouth dropped open. I cannot understate the power of seeing a part of my lived experience in someone else at that moment.

She acted as my first mentor, my first connection with the disabled community. What sacred conversations we had; for an hour a week we would put the world to rights. She was the first person to make me believe I could want more, that I deserved more as a disabled person. That I was enough, exactly as I am. Every time I said something that suggested an inner hatred, or expressed feelings of being a burden, doubting my worth, she would challenge me.

She ignited something in me, that would only grow.

I know the exact moment something in me snapped. It was in March 2020. I began to change for good after that.

I was a returning fourth-year medical student, scheduled for an advanced life support training session, and got there ten minutes late. I was nervous as I always was with such sessions after my injury. I worried I wouldn't be able to access things to help me, or in trying to get me access the organisers would make it a completely unrealistic scenario. I worried I'd just be in the way or somehow cause a scene.

I wheel up to the second floor and find some of my classmates waiting in the corridor. They tell me they've been split up into two groups because the instructors are concerned about Covid. I see the resuscitation instructor bustle towards us, on the phone to the organiser, clearly angry about the late start: 'This is the second time this has happened, and it's frankly ridiculous.'

Then her eyes fall on me, and I see her expression change, and I know she is about to seize an opportunity.

'. . . AND we have a lady in a WHEELCHAIR waiting in the corridor, so it's just unacceptable.'

She spits out the word wheelchair, as if saying a swear word.

I feel shaken, to be singled out in a crowd of peers I don't know well. I feel like nothing but a prop to her. She ends the call and the five of us file into the class-room. I start trying to tell her that I was perfectly fine waiting in the corridor, and that I was only there for a minute. She is clearly flustered, and mumbles something about how it was ridiculous while not looking at anyone directly. I tell her again clearly, trying to level my voice, that she didn't need to single me out, that everyone else was waiting too.

She bristles, leaves the room to get something and one of the other students leans over to me, telling me that it was good that I had said something.

I appreciate it, but I am still seething.

She comes back in and asks if everyone has signed the attendance sheet. I raise my hand and say I hadn't, yes me, the 'ONE IN THE WHEELCHAIR', using the same tone she had.

She winces at my words but gives the sheet to me silently.

I am aware of my body language. I try crossing my arms, and then decide to rest my elbows on the back of my back rest. I feel powerful.

For the first time since my injury, I get the impression that someone might be scared of me, and I realise that I don't have to meekly accept the treatment I receive. This gives me some fire; I feel alive, to be standing up for myself for the first time, in the face of the thousands of microaggressions that have been thrown at me.

I hadn't realised before that I may have this power – a power to demand better, to teach people and change how they go on to treat others.

I think about all the things I could say, deciding to ask her at the end why she felt she needed to single me out in front of the class, to use me as a token for her complaint. I wasn't scared or nervous – something had shifted. I felt adrenaline, I felt strong – this was all new. Things like this usually made me feel small, sad, defeated or mortified.

We go on break, and while others go to Costa I try to find a toilet I can fit into. I come back into the corridor and I see her. She walks by me, stepping away to avoid me. She hesitates, then turns around and says:

'Sorry – I'm really sorry, I didn't mean to be offensive, I'm sorry, it was just a stressful situation.'

I sit with her apology. I don't interrupt her ramble; I don't reassure her or try and stop her feeling bad. I let it reach its natural end and then I look at her directly in the eye and simply say, 'Okay.'

Who knew a word could feel so good? Not – 'No, no *I'm* sorry, *I'm* sorry', 'Don't worry about it', 'Thanks', or my usual attempts to minimise or brush things off. Just a simple . . . 'Okay'.

I have had hundreds of interactions far more grievous

than this one, but in that moment, I felt an anger that was powerful for the first time. It was not a hopeless anger.

I was so tired of trying to make other people feel better about the fact they had made me feel less than. I suddenly realised that this wasn't actually my job. Why should I be grateful when someone refuses to let me do something on my own? Why should I sit and listen to someone talking about my community in disparaging terms? Why should I let anyone talk over me? Why should I let anyone else define me?

People had been projecting their own ignorance on to me like a dirty stain. I stopped feeling like a victim once I decided to stop internalising these wounding reactions to me.

I was so tired of people assuming I must have an inner rage at the man that jumped and landed on me, when in fact I was so much angrier about how society treats disabled people, how people had treated me ever since I became a wheelchair user.

This new anger made me feel warm inside, rejuvenated, strong. Sadness and disappointment had been my prevailing emotions for such a long time; I found anger to be much more productive. It emboldened me, it felt warm, lit up my insides.

Sometimes frustration still overwhelms me. But anger I can cultivate. It grows into confidence, into boldness, into fearlessness, it makes me do things I never thought I could do. It makes me want to fight for change, for things to improve, for systems to change, and attitudes to shift.

Defining the boundaries of the things I will and will not accept has made me feel powerful.

I had spent the past year and a half feeling obliged to give up a part of me whenever I was asked by strangers what was wrong with me, what had happened to me, but I began to push back. *There's nothing wrong with me*, I try to reply with a smile now. If anything, I am reminding myself.

I have started to try and take control. I had worried that withholding this information would make people uncomfortable, overlooking the fact that they were the ones who had made me feel uncomfortable in the first place.

I still try hard to be understanding, empathetic, but as I am asked over and over the angrier I become. I am angry that disabled people must put up with this every day. We don't exist for this.

At first, I thought that as a disabled person I didn't carry much power or authority – learning how to do everything from scratch had stripped my confidence – but I began to recognise all the times when I do.

I can wheel into a room and my mere presence can make people stumble over their words, apologise for being too close to me, lose all composure, or say the most bizarre thing they can think of. I have power to make people feel uncomfortable. The power to make people honest.

I decided to stop shying away from it. I look, I *really* look at them.

'You seem uncomfortable.'

I have started calmly saying this to people, in the hope it will open up a different kind of conversation, to lead us somewhere different.

I've now learned to subvert or make these situations funny where I can – and so often they're absurd to begin with. One Friday night I was at the new pub by Farringdon Road, one of the cursed spots on the street, constantly changing hands. I was with Nathan and some friends, having just delivered takeaway to my parents' house as my dad was ill. (I was feeling so grateful for my motor attachment, allowing me not only independence but the ability to provide care for others when needed.)

I ordered some wine. There were three very drunk men on a table behind us. They looked mid-twenties. Loud, lairy. I had just witnessed one, who looked the drunkest, spill his goblet of gin and tonic twice, once over the table and then all over his trousers.

I attached my Batec handbike to go and ask the bartender if they had a ramp. I knew they had no ramp; I did this partly to remind them of this lack and partly to see if they would let us stay outside to finish our drinks after their curfew ended. As I was driving over, the gin-and-tonic soaked man let out two words:

'*VROOM VROOM!*'

I stopped, turned around and drove back to their table. I leant in, my face inches from his. I asked him to repeat what he just said. He suddenly was very quiet. His friends said, 'Don't worry, it's nothing.'

'Do you think that's funny?' I asked.

He was still looking down, and had gone red.

'Do you know what I thought was funny? When you spilled your entire drink down yourself. Now THAT really was funny.'

Who knows if these confrontations will make any difference, but I want to make him uncomfortable, through the power of sheer discomfort. Break the cycle, so someone else wouldn't have to hear it.

I have even begun to enjoy it! As someone whose need to please was once verging on pathological, it is liberating taking pleasure and power in something I used to find unbearable. Through embracing this discomfort I hope we can reach a place of deeper understanding, connection and empathy. Real change.

Where I once found staying silent or being polite was so much easier, taking charge of the conversation meant taking back some power.

To set boundaries for myself, to draw a line in the sand, I was getting angry enough to realise that I deserved to be treated better.

Doctor

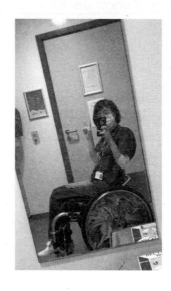

In 2021, I finally graduated and started work as a junior doctor in a busy central London hospital. It had taken a Herculean effort to get to this point and I was feeling confident, excited. But flashbacks hounded me in the first month. They were unexpected and visceral.

In my first week, as I spoke to a distressed patient who told me he didn't trust the night staff, I was swiftly plunged back to a night in Stanmore where I had felt so alone, so unsafe. I knew I had a urinary infection that night but had to repeatedly ask the new on-duty doctor for antibiotics. I remember crying in bed for hours until the pharmacist took charge and helped me.

Now, in my role as the doctor, I was constantly asking myself: is that patient's cubicle curtain closed? Does the patient know my name? Do they understand what's happening to them? Are they cold? Are they covered up? I was desperately trying to ensure that the wounding and humiliating things that had happened to me didn't happen to others.

On my first job, I saw a patient, G, who needed an endoscopy, a camera test that goes down the throat to get a biopsy, as her CT scan had showed something suspicious. On hearing the news, G's eyes fell and her chest sank visibly. It wasn't in fear of the possible malignancy, she told us. It was because of her husband. He'd been unwell before he died and had had an endoscopy at a different hospital to investigate the problem. She said he didn't get enough sedation and woke up while they were pushing the tube down his throat. He had flailed his arms and legs, in an attempt to get them to stop, but they had held him down and carried on. He had bruises all down one side of his body, and she said for the three years he lived after that he was never the same. I felt so strongly for this man, and his wife.

For a long time after my own hospital stay, I felt exactly like G's husband.

No evidence of PTSD was written in my notes by the cheerful inpatient psychologist who came to see me a few weeks post-injury. But the real trauma was yet to come. I still had two months in hospital to endure at that stage.

It's something I feel detached from now, like I am feeling sorry for a different girl.

But my body has held on to the memories longer than I have. For years, I've struggled with touch, my brain hard-wired to expect something horrible to happen, something painful, something shameful.

As a patient I once sat amid all of the kindness and all of the indignity, all of the beauty and all of the horror. Now, I feel more on the periphery, a secondary character rather than the protagonist. I bear witness to it all.

My experience now as a doctor has also been a strange reversal of everything I experienced as a patient: how little power I felt then, even as someone with some medical knowledge. How bewildering it was when people did not introduce themselves, explain what was going on; to feel no control over your own body, to feel completely at the whim of anonymous healthcare professionals.

At work I try to remember details from those months when I was an inpatient. As the years pass on it starts to feel like a lifetime ago, but I *want* to remember.

Every small act to protect my dignity, every time a nurse or doctor made the conscious effort to introduce themselves properly, to explain what was going on, to make me laugh, to reach out so I felt human in all of it. To cut through the smell of sterility, alcohol wipes and dressings.

I want to be that person for my patients, doing those small things that I appreciated so much in those hot, dark days. Someone holding out their hand to say hello, I see you, I know your name. Your name still belongs to you here. You're still a human being.

I joke that my time in hospital was the best placement I could have asked for to prepare me for being a doctor, but it's the truth.

Yet, even though I'm supposedly on the other side now, I still get the occasional reminder of how close I am to the line.

In the first hospital I worked, one of the perks was that I had access to the gigantic porters' lift. One morning I swiped my card and rolled in, distracted on my phone. The lift went up and opened on the eighth floor. I glanced up and saw a porter looking at me. He called to his colleague out of sight: 'There's a chair in here already, you can fit another one in.' I was confused, running that sentence over in my head while he got in with his colleague, who was pushing a patient, who was sitting in a wheelchair. I realised I hadn't pressed the button for the floor I was headed to.

'Where are you going? Oh, it looks like nowhere,' the porter said. I wanted to laugh at the gall of this man.

'I am not just a *chair*,' I managed to say.

The porter lost his composure. He was fiddling with the papers and the keys in his hands, as he embarked on a long-winded explanation about how that's what they refer to patients as when they're working.

'But no one should be called a chair,' I told him.

His colleague remarked, chuckling, that he was really stuck now.

He said he didn't want to say any more as he was digging himself a bigger hole. As we reached my floor and I wheeled out, I told him that was probably for the best.

I was used to being objectified by train and plane assistance staff, often called *a wheelchair* over walkie-talkies as they pull out ramps for me. But this was different, even if I could laugh about it later. I was at work! And in a hospital, where I thought I might be protected.

Other doctors may get misrepresented – sexist assumptions are still common on the wards, with female staff, particularly women of colour, assumed to be more junior than they are, or not believed to be the doctor in many cases. But no one else gets called a *chair*.

As a first- and second-year doctor I would move to a new job or 'rotation' every four months. Just as I was starting to get used to a place, or more importantly just as other people were getting used to me, I would be thrust into a new setting with strangers, and it would start all over again, as I shuttled through medicine, surgery, anaesthetics, general practice, A&E.

I felt pressure every time to make a good impression, as many colleagues had never worked with a wheelchair user before, and some acted like they had never even spoken to a wheelchair user who wasn't a patient.

On my second job, I was talking to my new registrar on a break after the ward round in the mess, and he began to tell me about his cousin's friend's neurological condition. He told me that it has meant 'he's now wheelchair-bound' and how sad it all was. I was stunned. So much so that I failed to say anything. I was confused as to whether he was aware who he was talking to. It made me wonder, who was I to him? To the rest of my colleagues?

Sometimes I felt as though I was seen as 'one of the good ones'; not *really* disabled. I was apart from fellow disabled people, singled out. Never seen as part of a community, a bigger group with a shared identity. I felt like I had slipped through the ranks, perhaps because I was still working. I wondered if this had anything to do with the tabloid myth of disabled scroungers – and the assumption that to be disabled meant to be out of work. To be a 'good' disabled person I had to keep up, not mention my needs, keep grafting, never complain.

I felt like an awkward hybrid, and in a system that so clearly demarcates the line between patient and doctor, this felt strange, wrong-footing.

When I was under investigations for persistent urinary infections, I would have to rip off my hospital bands as I rushed into another hospital to shadow a clinic. My realities were merging.

I spent my GP placement sympathising with patients who were waiting for referrals and results while fielding my own medical calls, chasing up my own appointments. I became accustomed to both.

It somehow challenged the old-fashioned division, the hierarchy.

I see how powerful this can be when a patient tells me how happy they are to see a doctor who is also a wheelchair user; how much it has comforted them.

Younger people reach out to me on social media, people who were told they could not be a doctor as a wheelchair user by a teacher, occupational health staff or some other figure of authority, so they did not apply. If they had never seen one before, who are they to dispute this?

It made me realise that I must be visible. I am not doing it just for me any more. I need to be in these spaces. To fight my way into these rooms.

There are so many moments of connection now, big and small. When a patient with a brain injury jokes to me that he sets off all the alarms in airport security, because he has a metal plate in his head, I say, me too, because of the rods in my spine. He smiles.

Me too.

It's so powerful not to feel alone in illness or in managing a long-term condition or disability.

A patient who uses an electric wheelchair tells me that my foot has got caught behind my footplate while I am listening to her chest; she knows all about it, because it happens to her too. She says she can't describe to me how good it is to see a disabled doctor.

One day, I read in the notes that the woman I am about to see, S, has a learning disability and hates being in hospital, but I see her face light up when I enter the room: 'I was in a wheelchair before!!' she shouts. There is an understanding that we share, a level of trust already in place, which I did not have to build. An infrastructure of deep recognition.

The next time I see S is a year later during a night shift; she looks like she has had a fall this time, blood down her face and she's wearing pyjamas. I don't think she will remember me from so long ago. All of a sudden, she puts her hand on my head, and then kneels down to lean on me. She tells me she wants me to treat her, and she shows me pictures of her family. I am so touched by this.

I am more like you than you know, I want to tell these people, but they seem to understand it implicitly.

And I was emboldened as I met more and more people like me. I was working on the admissions unit when I realised the blind man that was walking around the ward wore a lanyard, suggesting he was a staff member. I was surprised by my excitement, by my urge to go and speak to him, to tell him what it meant to me that he was also here. Our experiences may have been vastly different, but I suddenly did not feel like the only one.

Ironically, despite the challenges, most of the time in the hospital I feel in perfect synchrony with my wheelchair. I can be swift and nimble moving through corridors, turning sharply, gliding down slopes, knowing when to lean, when to push one wheel with more force, or that when I bend over my right wheel my left hand instinctively catches my left push rim to lift myself up. The wheels and metal below me are an extension of my being. Multiple steps have developed into a seamless movement, so much so that it has become fun.

My favourite is the slope from the doctors' mess down to the main lifts of the hospital. It is the steepest decline in the building. On night shifts I would close my eyes for a few seconds and lift my hands off my push rims, feeling the rush of air past my face. Hurtling down into blackness while feeling in complete control.

When faced with the disarray around a patient's bed, the awkward side table that's taller than me and usually has tiny wheels that only go in one direction, I have had to find workarounds. Learn how to dodge an observation trolley with wires hanging off it on the floor. An oxygen tank with a tube dangling down, which I have to try to avoid rolling over. Or my personal nemesis: a pair of patient's slippers.

And certain opportunities have come with my new status. Ahead of a thirteen-hour shift in the admissions ward, I arrived and noticed police milling around, hands resting on their vests, looking out of place. Nurses in red uniforms, signalling that they were part of the critical response team, were everywhere.

You can usually tell how the day will go by the state of the corridor in the morning. An older woman was walking around, shouting that she's supposed to get on a plane today, while a resigned-looking healthcare worker followed her. There was a man with a similar entourage in the opposite room, a man who had tried everything he could to hurt himself. I watched him being ushered back to his own room.

Then two crash calls came in, one after the other: a possible allergic reaction to contrast dye injected for an MRI scan and a visitor who had collapsed in the main reception with a seizure.

I heard my red bleep buzz excitedly.

This is a peri arrest on floor 4 East wing, I repeat this is a peri arrest on floor 4 East wing.

I started to make my way from the ward and noticed immediately that there was a 'situation' unfolding in reception. Ten people in red uniforms, police officers, mental health nurses and healthcare assistants were standing around a patient who I later learned had been sectioned.

She was wearing her own clothes on top of a patient gown, sitting in her wheelchair. Staff were attempting to stop her from leaving in case she hurt herself.

She screamed at anyone who tried to touch her. I didn't see this situation progressing well. Crowding around a patient never helps.

I saw her start to wheel towards the back exit of the ward, so I wheeled myself between her and the door, unsure if this was the right thing to do but I did it anyway, so there might be time for staff members to persuade her to stay voluntarily.

She looked at me and stopped shouting.

I was not an aggressor in this situation; perhaps I was a distraction more than anything. I waited there so they were able speak to her for a few minutes, explain what was going on. The nursing team came up to me afterwards to tell me how helpful that was. Perhaps feeling as though I'm in the way can be a good thing sometimes.

People are not expecting me here – and that can disrupt the course of events, diffuse the day-to-day dramas of a busy hospital. I am out of the ordinary. It can be enough to cut through the tension.

I don't want to be naive; I am sure on the wrong day, in the wrong place, I am just as at risk of being assaulted as other colleagues, who I've seen bearing the brunt of a patient's frustration and rage. But there is something about the introduction of the wheelchair that makes people pause. I hold power because I am never seen as threatening. I hold power because I am underestimated. People don't quite know what to do with me, which can work in my favour.

In many instances I have lowered the heat of a situation with an aggressive patient or family member simply by being present. I have learned that I have the ability to neutralise, to de-escalate. That it's not just physical strength that allows you to be in control of a situation.

But how much power I'm granted now fluctuates dramatically according to the setting I'm in. I can hold a lot of power in the clinic room. I am listened to. As soon as I take my stethoscope and lanyard off and leave work, I become both hypervisible and utterly ignored. I realise I have been given privileges because of my job that other disabled people do not have. I fluctuate between having a huge amount of responsibility at work, and then leave and am assumed to have none at all. It is a jarring transition.

Colleagues often say they hate wearing their lanyard and stethoscope outside of work, but I am hesitant to rid myself of one of the only identifiers that earns me respect and status outside the hospital. I live in absolutes of being either a care giver or a care receiver, and there is a power imbalance that comes with this.

I spend my life navigating these vast shifts of responsibility. Writing a person's name down for the last time on their death certificate, then unable to open the heavy door to leave the office.

I am frequently grateful that my injury can put me on more of an equal footing with patients, and for the advantages this brings with it. It helps that I am often literally at eye level to people lying or sitting down.

I see other doctors who cannot help but loom over patients in bed. Very tall consultants struggle to shorten their frame by bending, kneeling and still end up towering over someone. I do not have to worry about this added power dynamic, the physically underlined hierarchy. It can allow for more collaboration, for a real partnership.

My experience with patients has changed since my injury. There is an openness, an eagerness to connect with me that wasn't so present before. My wheelchair acts as a visible scar; I have clearly been on their side of the hospital bed before. There are, of course, other doctors who have been much sicker than me, through chronic illness or other circumstances, but I am *visibly* a previous patient.

My baseline as a patient was that I wanted to feel seen and to feel heard. I believe this is what we all want. *A Fortunate Man*, John Berger's account of the life of a country doctor in the sixties, is still, to me, one of the most accurate portraits of medicine. He so beautifully describes how patients want to know that their illness exists outside of themselves, that they are not alone in their suffering.

Equally, disabled patients want to see their experiences too – and they can when visibly disabled healthcare workers are around them. I know how precious and rare that feeling is, when you live in a body that is not well represented in the world. There is something so special about finding a piece of your life in someone else.

On my anaesthetics job I felt privileged to care for patients as they fell asleep. One particular patient stays in my mind. M was lying in a hospital bed, but even so I could see that he was a tall man; I imagined he would usually command a room when he walked in.

As I go through the pre-operative checklist, I have learned to ask patients about their favourite food, their favourite holiday, in the hopes they will then dream of it. M tells me about his recent trip to Gran Canaria, and the terrapins and the banana trees he saw. It's only when I am about to put the oxygen mask over his nose and mouth that he tells me that he is afraid. One tear escapes from his left eye and I catch it with my finger.

His voice is muffled under the mask I hold tightly to his face to avoid leaks. I hold the side of his face, not only to secure his mask, but in an attempt to steady him.

His operation will be major, life-changing. He will wake up different, I know it.

He starts to tell me how the terrapins are different from the turtles but trails off—

He is asleep; we have pushed him into that state where he will remain for the next six hours. I hope he dreams of sunshine and terrapins and banana trees. I wipe away the single tear that has fallen down his face. You are giving your body to us for the next few hours. We are in charge now, I think, as the anaesthetist supervises me to tilt his head back to push the tube down his throat, then thread a wire into his artery.

I think back to my time in a room like this, in a bed like this. How for everyone else around me it was just another normal day at work. I'm glad I can remember that for this man, for every patient who comes to us, this is so far from normal, and how much they need us to hold them through it. I am glad I can't remember how this metal instrument was also used to open up my own throat, scratching the roof of my mouth, the tube pushed down into my trachea. The blood from my mouth and from my wrists. But I remember what I needed to from those moments. There is a certain surreal quality in the fact I am doing to others what was done to me.

In medicine the line between tenderness and brutality is paper-thin and crossed so quickly. Between the barbaric and the beautiful. This is where the full expanse of life occurs. I find this as a doctor daily. One minute I may be witnessing a man in his dying moments on Boxing Day, blood smeared down a hospital gown; the next I might encounter an elderly lady who is trying to tip me for looking after her by shakily pressing a £10 note into my hand.

Sometimes I feel I am verging into the more brutal territory; for instance, when I am trying to place a fifth cannula in an elderly patient who doesn't understand what is happening and keeps pulling them out, her arms a deep purple with bruising from previous attempts. She's telling me she just wants someone to look after her. Understandably she does not realise that is what I am trying to do.

When I see a children's drawing of red and orange shapes that has been taped to the wall opposite a dying man's bed, I wonder if he saw those shapes before he died, or if he was just trying to breathe.

But there is joy, absurdity, when I am racing a wheelchair-using seven-year-old down the corridor of the paediatric department. A kitchen utensil on an X-ray inserted where it shouldn't be. Camaraderie with colleagues all working together through the night.

Moment after moment strung together to form a thirteen-hour shift. When I get to the end I barely remember the moments that made me nearly cry, that made my heart jump, that made me shake, that made me laugh. But I want to remember the moments that matter. I do not want them to be lost in the blur of an on-call shift. Constantly moving forward, on to the next patient, on to the next plan.

I want to remember when I could do good, make someone feel better, no matter how briefly. A smile, a sigh of relief, helping them to get home.

At first, I did not want my injury and hospital stay to change me, but of course, it did. It continues to change me, for good and bad. One thing I will never regret is how it taught me to hold dignity and autonomy above all else.

It is getting easier now, to draw the line between my past and my present. It helps that I get to go home at the end of the day. It is strange that I'm starting to feel so comfortable in hospital again, when it was once my nightmare.

I still have flashbacks often though. Perhaps I always will.

I see a patient make seemingly irrational demands and I instinctively recognise the visceral feeling of losing control, the pure frustration. The attempt to grasp at strands of autonomy. How I once raged against the over-sized pills I had to take and refused to swallow them.

I know how important minuscule things become,

when you're going through the inexplicable experience of being an inpatient for months on end.

When I notice the two patients who have been causing mayhem on the ward become co-conspirators, starting to speak in hushed tones and giggling, walking off arm in arm, I think of Rubes and me gossiping about staff and patients, racing down corridors at 1 a.m., throwing tennis balls up and down the length of the ward.

I don't think knowing this necessarily makes you a better doctor, but I know for me it helps. I am grateful for this understanding.

I remember sitting in an endocrine clinic. The patient had sheepishly told the consultant that she had not been taking her medication for her thyroid because it tasted horrible. The consultant was confused and didn't understand. I could empathise with the patient; I had been on the same medication, and it was like eating salt. This small encounter stayed with me. This consultant knew so much about the molecular mechanism, the research, the impact of this tiny tablet, but not how it feels in your mouth.

I am glad it's me who's on duty when certain people come in. I am glad whenever I can care for a patient who also has a spinal cord injury. Who has a mobility aid. Or who is fed up with being in hospital, who is tired, crying – or tired of crying.

One after another I meet these patients and we share a connection, and I am glad each time that I dragged myself to work and feel in control, like I can make an impact. I feel equipped. I know that these patients will feel better after talking to me. I know that these patients won't experience the added injury of a hurtful or ignorant comment. I hope they will feel safe with me.

I know what it's like to be lying in that hospital bed, and how easy it would be for me to get there again. What little could lead me there.

It is almost inevitable that I will have a hospital stay at some point in my life for my spinal cord injury, but other doctors in my cohort, in their mid-twenties, would rarely expect hospitalisation or procedures in such a definitive way.

I realise that I can bridge the gap. I can be both, and neither one nor the other. There can be a dynamic relationship between my two identities. I can break down the binary between doctor and patient and how healing this can be. I can continue to navigate the messiness of multiple identities, to accept these blurred lines.

All the signs that I don't belong in this field make me even more adamant that I do.

Normal

Many of the ways in which I function would not be considered 'normal' now.

I don't even function as other disabled people do because disability is characterised by such a diversity, a vastness of experience. I cannot google why my neuropathic pain feels different than usual, why my leg is kicking out in a certain way, why my foot is twitching as I go to sleep. We are the only experts in our own bodies.

My body speaks a different language that I have had to learn through the dictionary of experience. A certain spasm in my leg will tell me I need to pee, that I have cut my foot, that I might have a UTI. I must scan through my own recent past to be able to interpret the signs.

I quickly discovered the many ways disabled people adapt and flex to do daily tasks, depending on the person, the injury, the sensation, the power – what works for them. I was beginning to appreciate the seemingly endless capacity to adapt, to develop new ways of doing things. However, it often feels like these adaptations are pathologised, rather than valued or celebrated, reflecting the language we use, or avoid using.

The way I open doors, prop myself up on my elbows, hold one of my wheels while I reach down to pick something up might look unnatural to others but has become second nature to me, and works just fine.

So often, the things I do are interpreted in relation to my disability, and my perceived health needs. I once mentioned how much I liked swimming to a GP I was working with. Ah yes, *swimming for physio*, she repeated and proceeded to say it three times in the conversation. I wanted to interrupt her: no I do swimming for FUN! Is that allowed? It's as if my body is now a never-ending improvement project, rather than a source of joy, experience, living.

Society loves a binary, and disability cannot fit neatly into it; we don't see that disability is another, equally valid way of existing, rather than a perpetual state of sickness or defectiveness. In the same way, there is little understanding of how disability might fluctuate: if you are an ambulatory wheelchair user who can sometimes walk, or if you are chronically ill and may have days of high or low energy. There is no space given for the fluidity and flux, and for the inevitable ups and downs of living in a disabled body.

I learned how vast the variety of the disabled experience is, and how little of this the world acknowledges.

The lens through which I previously viewed disability and illness was very likely coloured by the language I had grown up hearing. Language I still hear now at work, which is used to describe others and can now be used to describe me. Objectification, passivity and ideas of tragedy are perpetuated. Medical terms seep into the perceptions of disability, and how it's treated in much broader contexts. The whole idea of normality has permeated so much of how we live and what we believe.

There is a certain passivity in the language used to describe me and others like me. 'Wheelchair-bound' makes me want to grind my teeth, yet it is so pervasive. It completely negates the idea that this wheelchair is a tool for my mobility, for my independence. What does it even mean? It all suggests something static. To be bound. To be tied down. To be imprisoned. To be lower than others. To have less freedom than others. No other mobility device is described like this. The wheelchair symbol is an omen, an imagined future, a terrifying prospect.

If someone describes me as wheelchair-bound, they are denying my reality.

As a doctor I have sat in discussions with consultants and physiotherapists where they talk about whether a patient is 'confined to a wheelchair' at a baseline or not. They may not mean to do it, but their language suggests this patient is done for before they've even begun, that there's no need for rehab or physio.

This damaging undercurrent applies to so much of the language we use. *Special needs.* No one has *special* needs. Everyone has access needs. Is using glasses a special need? Describing it as 'special' makes it clear that these adaptations and accommodations are not a given, that we should be grateful any time our basic needs are met. There is nothing special about needing the bathroom.

The 'special' provisions I'm granted, e.g. skipping the queues at airports, feel like a pittance against the indignity of flying as a wheelchair user, terrified my wheelchair will break in the hold, unable to use the toilet on most planes. It's hard enough just to catch a train! I receive the best and the worst: moments of such kindness from staff and others when they help me and let me sit in first class. But then I'm left stranded, hurtling away from my destination when no one comes to help me off at my stop.

The same linguistic gymnastics are applied to the very word 'disabled'. A psychiatrist on my first placement back at medical school called the toilet a disabled toilet and then quickly apologised to me, as if hearing the word itself would offend me. If a health professional is *apologising* for my label, then where does that leave me?

This only underlines that there's something about me that is missing, inept, shameful.

I found this early in my injury when I was still at Stanmore and a fellow patient's husband wouldn't stop explicitly telling me how sorry he felt for me in the break room. It wouldn't be the first time I'd hear this. No wonder this pity is so pervasive, considering how we talk about all these issues, the language we've inherited.

Maybe I could understand a pitying reaction better when I was still stuck in hospital, but it continued to crop up, even once I was out in the world, doing a dream job that I had worked so hard for, beginning to enjoy life again, and feeling more capable every day in my new body.

Strangers will look at me with pity as if from one glance they can understand my life as a whole. Some people are compelled to approach me to tell me just how bad they feel for me. This might happen at the supermarket, or when I am out with friends, or even at work.

It always feels as though they have forced their way into my world and spat on it. In their minds, what has happened to me is a tragedy, end of story.

I might be confronted with the phrase 'Oh isn't it awful being in a wheelchair?', no matter what I am doing at the time. As if you'd ever go up to an elderly person in public and say, 'Isn't it awful being old? I knew someone who was old once, and God it just looks dreadful! How do you cope with being so old?'

I am reminded of the gap between my perceived reality and the reality others project on to visible disability. Often it feels like nothing I say or do in the moment can persuade anyone otherwise. It is assumed that, more than anything, I must wish for a cure for my supposed affliction but will bravely go forward with my smaller life.

Hand in hand with this, there is a pressure now that I must do something extraordinary that proves I still have value in society. Maybe I should be in the Paralympics or accomplish some other epic physical feat. It must be something grand. I must *overcome* my disability, be tragically triumphant. There is no space for mediocrity here.

I was once part of a television show, and the blurb described me as 'a practising Junior Doctor in a busy London A&E department, refusing to let her wheelchair stand in her way to fulfilling her dreams'. I laughed out loud. Ignoring the clumsy oxymoron of a wheelchair standing, this statement is ridiculous to me. I owe everything to my wheelchair; it is the reason I am able to do any of this! Yet it is seen as a barrier to overcome.

The only thing standing in my way is usually an oblivious person as I try to get past them. It reminds me of the military language pervasive in cancer diagnoses; battles that are 'won' or 'lost'. Again, it individualises, making it somehow seem like it all boils down to a personal problem, an individual tragedy or failure.

I am seen as in a state of perpetual acuity, as if this has always only *just* happened to me. As if I have not grown, could not have recovered at all, stuck in a state of shock.

The first time an old schoolfriend met me after my injury she told me she would have killed herself if it had happened to her – so casually I felt as if I were imagining it. She said it as if it were a fact of life. When I am faced with a strange question or comment like this I am taken aback, often because I have forgotten how I am perceived until that moment.

It is an uphill battle to defend my happiness, my quality of life to strangers, and I kick myself whenever I resort to such a useless exercise. 'I am doing well!! I promise!' I put on my best smile, but it doesn't seem to convince them.

These assumptions of tragedy are not preconceptions that individuals have plucked from thin air. There is an undercurrent, running through everything we watch and read, everything we're exposed to. The very language we're born into. It is so insidious, and I only started looking at it critically after my injury.

The film *Me Before You*, a (now controversial) romantic drama, depicts a man with a high-level spinal cord injury, played by Sam Claflin (who, of course, does not have this disability), who falls in love with his caregiver, Emilia

Clarke. They have a brief romance, and at the end of the film he travels to Switzerland to undergo an assisted suicide.

Watching it before my injury I didn't take a second to question the plot. All the characters accept it too. He must want to die: what else is here for him in this body? A beautiful girlfriend? A loving family? An enormous house? Of course, he wants to end it, because a life in his state is not a life worth living.

There is a viral photo that floats around the internet; whenever I see it, it fills me with discomfort. It is a picture of a child's headstone in a cemetery. On his headstone is a sculpture of a wheelchair, and a boy standing up out of it, reaching upwards, leaving it behind.

The articles usually share it with a caption that suggests that he can finally be at peace, 'liberated from the device'. I don't know anything about this family, or the reasons they chose this image, but it is often co-opted to support the view that disability is suffering, and death is the only release. I guess heaven isn't accessible either.

I have to be careful about what I see on social media. I can very easily come across a comment that devalues my entire existence. A post that implies it would be better if I didn't exist, that I am a drain on resources, that I should be grateful for the bare minimum, that I am a burden.

How many times have I gone to binge an old television series or comfort-watch that I remember from my childhood like *Law & Order*, and it's an episode about a woman who killed her disabled son because she didn't want him to suffer. I can't catch a break!

When I think of these examples from books, film and

television, who can blame strangers on the street for their poorly chosen words to me? They are just expressing a wider narrative our society drills into us.

No matter how much I speak about my recovery, my joy, my acceptance of my injury, I get online comments insisting that I'm pretending, that deep down I won't ever be able to move on from this, that my life is destroyed, and I am in denial. *Life in a wheelchair means life in prison* is a phrase I still remember from an article written about my injury.

It is very hard to try to see a future for yourself when everyone is telling you otherwise, when no one will believe what you say about yourself. *Poor brave tragic girl.*

I have experienced such anger and suspicion whenever I have strayed from the dominant and somehow acceptable narrative of disability as something sad and pitiful, or strayed from a position of gratitude. I started to realise that people do not like challenge – or to have to change their ingrained opinions.

No matter how eloquent or clear I could be about what happened and my life now, there will always be people who see my life as nothing but a struggle.

Accepting this was slow and hard, but it liberated me. I began to realise that my quality of life is entirely unrelated to the projections of other people, or the terms they use to define me. I started to realise that these narratives, and therefore my body, on some level exist to make able-bodied people feel better about themselves. If I'm not as miserable as I'm expected to be it seems to make some people uncomfortable; they'd like to be able to look down on me. If I don't play along, where does that leave them? We all need stories that make us feel good about ourselves. My therapist even jokes that, as disabled people, it is our unpaid job to make able-bodied people feel better.

A disabled friend told me that while volunteering at her local food bank, a man using the service started chatting to her, but once he realised that she was there to give food rather than receive it, he became angry and refused to take anything from her.

A man I shared a lift with once cried in shame on hearing that I had a job and he didn't.

There was a patient, X, who I often saw during a job in A&E; he would come in every week or so. He was someone we'd refer to as a 'frequent flyer' to the department, flitting between majors and minors depending on the severity of week he was having. He was usually drunk, sometimes angry, sometimes on the floor, sometimes unconscious.

One day I was clerking him (likely the tenth time I'd seen him come in) and he was semi-sober. He asked me why I was using a wheelchair. I told him I didn't have time to go into it, as I had so many other patients waiting, but he seemed desperate for some connection.

I told him what happened to me, but also stressed that I was doing well. He seemed upset, unnerved by my last comment. 'How can you possibly live like that?' he asked. He turned over, not wanting to speak to me any longer.

I looked at him wide-eyed.

*

These are a handful of stories from hundreds of interactions I have had with people over the years since my injury, that show me the warped and conflicting messaging tied to disability. People may hear what I say, but they cannot believe it; it is a contradiction to everything they have been told before.

The pity people project on to me, just by looking at me, calls back to the outdated, charity model of disability, which is much like the medical model, in terms of viewing us as victims, the objects of pity. But it also implies that disabled people should rely on charitable causes and be the receivers (never the givers) of services.

I have a complex relationship with charity. It can do such good when services are missing from the NHS, from social care, but in the world that I hope for, disabled people shouldn't have to rely on charity. It upholds an archaic infrastructure that we must beg for support, always be in need, always be the grateful recipients.

How many charity events have I been to, holding champagne while strangers peer down at me, or lean, hands on their knees, looking at me sadly? In my experience these spaces can make people feel much more comfortable with asking intrusive questions or making outrageous comments. Charity can do so much good, but not when it reinforces the harmful archetypes of disability.

I was invited to speak at a sports quiz for a spinal injury charity soon after my discharge, to talk about what help I had received. It took a while to dawn on me that I was the only one present with a spinal injury. I felt I was invited to be gawked at, paraded out. One of the staff members was amazed Nathan had stayed with me after my injury.

It made me realise how crucial disabled input and representation is in these spaces; if disabled people are not an integral part of these organisations, how wrong they can go.

I became a trustee of the spinal cord injury charity Back Up, which had given me advice early on in my injury. I was wary after my prior experiences but at Back Up, I look around the room during trustee meetings and half the people have spinal cord injuries. I feel we are talking about the right things, with the right people, and so much good can be done.

Inspiration porn is a phrase coined by Stella Young, the late disabled activist, that I first heard in her brilliant TED talk. Our disabled lives are presumed to be horrendous, a daily horror show, but also somehow inspirational, incredible. The fact that I have merely dragged myself out of bed is a triumph in itself.

The first time a stranger called me an inspiration for being at the gym it completely threw me. My mere presence in the place was amazing to him. I have heard the word 'inspiring' so often now it has lost all meaning. I cringe at its sound, even when well intended. It has become an empty platitude. What am I inspiring you to do? I want to know. Often there is no clear answer; it's hard to pin down. Am I inspiring you to advocate for disabled people? To campaign for accessible places? Or am I really just making you feel good about yourself?

I remember finding it particularly ridiculous right at the start when I was first injured. Everyone was telling me how inspiring I was, when it was a time I had never needed inspiration more.

I yearn for more neutrality in how we think and talk about disability. If society didn't celebrate, but neutralised and normalised disability, would an injury like mine feel so obliterating? Such a gutting experience? It is hard to even imagine that reality.

Instead, I am simultaneously special, inspiring and possess superpowers, while leading a sad, pitiful, small life.

We are starved of neutral imagery and ordinary stories of disabled people. When I came out of hospital, I longed to see disabled people just getting on with life.

I realised that the 'superhero' narrative so often placed on disabled people is also placed on doctors and all healthcare workers, too. It's a useful narrative, politically, as it individualises our struggle, takes us out of the societal and political context, putting the onus on us as people to live up to these impossible ideals.

In hospital, I get abuse, platitudes and praise for being a disabled doctor, but it sometimes feels as though I'm never treated like a human being. We are put on a pedestal built by others, which perpetuates the same old narratives rather than approaching disability with open eyes and open ears.

We need our own voices to be heard when trying to make real change.

PART 4:
Reflections on life today

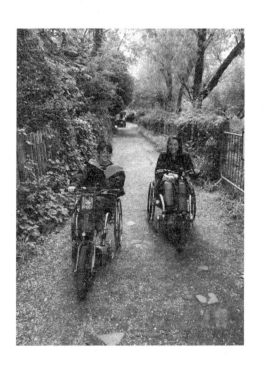

Those who have come before me

It has been years now – what feels like a lifetime – since my injury.

So much has happened.

I sometimes wonder to myself: how on earth did I get here? To a place of acceptance, of joy, with a sense of a security in my new state?

It didn't all come from me. It began with surrounding myself with the right people. Finding power in a community, finding power in shared knowledge and learning.

When I got out of hospital finding other people like me was so important. I had been thrust out into a foreign world with no map, and no one to talk to that looked like I did now. Where did I belong? Who else was going through this, or had come out the other side?

Suddenly I was experiencing something completely alien, something my friends and family had no background in. I felt so alone in navigating this new life. I would scroll through Instagram, following every wheelchair user I could find, desperate to see people who shared some experiences with me.

I still felt lost and bewildered by so many questions around how to live my life in this new context. I had a thousand urgent practical questions, as well as many much more abstract ones.

So I began the only way I knew how – by gathering knowledge. The beauty of the internet became clear: it was a landscape of advice that made it easy to connect with others, hundreds of miles away.

Watching YouTube videos of a stranger in America showing how they transfer into a car, talking in detail about which catheters they use, how they get into the bath. (I hadn't known that was even possible!) I spent hours taking in these videos, instructing viewers on every physical activity you could possibly imagine, none of which I'd ever given a second thought to in my old life. I felt oddly connected to these strangers across the world videoing themselves in their bathrooms, while I watched from mine.

A few months after I was discharged, I took part in a sports weekend specially organised for newly injured people, run by Stoke Mandeville Hospital, a spinal unit where the Paralympics movement was born, with the first Stoke Mandeville Games coinciding with the opening ceremony of the 1948 London Olympics.

I hated the team sports but enjoyed the swimming, although what I could do in the pool would have been more accurately described as 'flailing around'. It was an encouraging environment, all the other recently injured people cheering me on from the sidelines, including Rubes. I didn't care that I came last.

It was my first trip without Nathan, and I had just

been switched to a new drug to try and reduce my leg spasms, but which had somehow only made them worse. I felt them actively fighting against me whenever I moved.

I had a panic attack on the first night, my body an unruly toddler I had been left in sole charge of, without a clue how to look after it.

But among the stress of battling with my changed body, I met some great people who were also new to this life. We talked about the dearth of information available once you were discharged, our experiences in rehab, how difficult it was to transition back into the outside world. We felt like other newly injured people might find these conversations helpful too, so six of us embarked on making a podcast. We spoke about the challenges of adjusting to discharge, of parenting with a disability, sex, relationships, continence, access – everything and anything.

For me, sitting in a room with five other disabled people every month, a space to share our challenges, our fears, our laughs, did big things for my confidence and for my sense of self.

Then Covid hit, and we had to move it online. Ironically, this opened up a bigger world: I suddenly had an excuse to reach out to a huge variety of people with spinal cord injuries, whose journeys I had been following online.

I was able to talk on Zoom with pro surfers, models, dancers, therapists, television presenters, artists, mouth painters, photographers, writers, travellers. A diverse, flawed, brilliant crew. Most of all, *interesting* people leading *joyful* lives, accepting themselves as they were, while rejecting the societal constraints and barriers built by others.

Want to get in the sea? Want to live in a camper van? Want to be the first person to do XYZ? They were going to find a way.

Basically, they were doing whatever the fuck they wanted to do.

Where had they all been hiding? Or was I just not looking for them before? The lives they were living were a long way from the static categories and diagnostic numbers I'd fixated on in hospital. They were simply living. Rich lives, good lives. They had found their place in the world. They described experiences, jobs and lives that still felt incomprehensible to me as a newly injured person.

I spent hours in phone calls and video conversations with people I had never met face to face, but immediately felt I could talk to about intimate things, sharing things that might take me years to open up about with others.

I learned so much, particularly from meeting and hearing from disabled people who were disabled from birth or childhood. In my experience they can be hardier, unflinching. Perhaps they have had to maintain a sense of self-worth through much more.

I was beginning to feel proud to share a bond and an experience with these people. Nowadays, I seek out my disabled community whenever I get the chance. Through WhatsApp groups we share tips and advice; we rant, we vent.

An appreciation of kinship was forming in my mind, in all aspects of my life. I was finding strength in numbers.

*

Vince and I kept in touch after being discharged from Stanmore. These days, we call each other every other day, or every day if he's sick, or in hospital. He remembers everything about my life: he'll say, you sounded angry about your friend three weeks ago, how are you doing with them now? How was your appointment, did work go okay?

Vince, in his late forties, was a scaffolder in Essex before we met at Stanmore. Our paths would almost certainly never have crossed. He always greets me on the phone with a Hello best friend! Hello lovely one, Good morning my little buddy, princess, my favourite person, trouble, my dance partner . . .

I talk to him more than I do to most people in my life.

'We've got to get this wedding organised, bubba!' he tells me, after I announce that Nathan and I are engaged.

It is funny to feel such an instant closeness. We may have acquired our disabilities or been born with them, but either way, these people feel like family.

I was told early on in my hospital stay by a fellow patient that, by sustaining spinal cord injuries, we had joined a 'club that no one wants to be a part of'. That's how I felt at the start, before I realised that the *club* is one of the great parts. Some of the best people I have met are disabled, have spinal cord injuries. Sure, the injury can be hard, but the people? The people are brilliant.

Often, when I pass another wheelchair user in the street, we share a nod or smile. It feels as though we know each other already in some small way.

I have found a place in this group.

A girl called Katie messaged me on Instagram asking

for some advice on something she had heard on the podcast. She was injured the year after me. We end up seeing each other every so often, whenever I go up to Scotland or she's down in London.

I met up with her in Edinburgh, after a week-long conference in Glasgow, and we went on a cycle with our handbikes. We got to a park hut and she taught me how to lean back on a wall, by back-wheel balancing, inching backwards to rest against it. We hung out in the meadows, watching some fire dancers practise and eating pizza.

It was the first time I had felt at ease on the trip, that I could breathe out. I didn't know how to tell her how happy I was to see her, to see someone like me. I didn't have to keep up any pretence that I wasn't exhausted, that I wasn't in pain, that I wasn't frustrated it took me an hour to find an accessible toilet earlier that day; she understood it all already.

She told me how she's trying to get Edinburgh council to fund her climbing equipment so she can get up some trees again. I love her.

We spent New Year's together the following year, and it was such a joy to introduce her to my friends. I am so proud. This is my community.

Around the same time that I was meeting and speaking with more and more disabled people, I started reading. A good friend who lends books like he's paid to do it passed me one he thought would interest me. It was called *Nothing About Us Without Us: Disability Oppression and Empowerment* by James Charlton. I had read nothing on disability before then. When I read the line,

'We know that when a person becomes disabled, she or he immediately becomes "less",' I was shocked. No one had said it aloud before, but it was true. It was what I was experiencing. It was as if everyone was pretending otherwise, but it was what I felt every day. There was no sugar coating, no faux inspiration to be found in these pages. Instead, I learned about the disability justice movement, the Americans with Disabilities Act, how different countries and cultures perceived disability, how the fight against injustice continues today.

It was a short but powerful read and my first step to realising I could be a part of something much greater than just my personal struggle.

Soon after, I read *Disability Visibility*, an anthology of stories from many different disabled people, curated by Alice Wong, which revealed to me the vast expanse of experiences.

I watched *Crip Camp*, a documentary about young disabled people at a summer camp in America in the seventies. Many went on to fight for the kinds of access enshrined in law now.

I saw amazing images of the Capitol Crawl in 1990, where 200 disabled people crawled up the steps of the Capitol to protest inaccessible design, part of a demonstration which led to the Americans with Disabilities Act.

I learned how disabled people have led the way for around a hundred years in campaigning for rights, on the streets and lobbying the Houses of Parliament and making political change happen across the world. How, in the UK, a disabled workers' union, the National League of the Blind, marched to a rally in London in

1920, to demand better working conditions and pay, and in so doing paved the way for the Jarrow March and the powerful workers' movements that later emerged. How in the seventies disabled campaigners fought for rights on public transport, and in the eighties campaigned for anti-discrimination legislation.

I learned about DAN, the Disabled People's Direct Action Network, and their campaigns of non-violent civil disobedience in the nineties. The long hard road to getting the 1995 Disability Discrimination Act in place.

I learned about the birth of eugenics, and the Nazi Aktion T4 programme, with its ideas of 'life unworthy of life'. I read Harriet McBryde Johnson's essay 'Unspeakable Conversations' on having to debate with Professor Peter Singer on her right to exist.

I was realising how expendable our lives were to others.

I read Frances Ryan's book *Crippled*, on the decimation of the social care system in the UK, and I saw myself in real time, through the Covid pandemic, how disabled people were left to die and forgotten about, collateral damage, brushed aside. I saw how our lives matter less, in every reference to 'underlying health conditions'.

I began to question the figures of authority that were describing disabled people. I began to interpret the language of eugenics.

I read about disability theory, learned academic language, realised that people had been studying this for decades.

I learned about England's history with a fascination with bodies deemed different in freak shows, and how that fascination has endured to today in different forms. That for centuries we have been hidden away or put out on display on the whim of others' aversion or curiosity.

I learned about the long history of disabled people, across the spectrum, and how it has left us with the cultural legacy and stereotypes that I was experiencing myself. I was learning that we have always been here.

I learned how activists and pioneering thinkers today are dismantling ideas like productivity and normality, to reinsert disabled people into the spaces that have excluded and erased us.

I began to see how this all related to me. I was realising that I belonged to a culture. I was beginning to understand the work that thousands and thousands of disabled people before me had done, for me to be able to live the life I do now.

I devoured books – scribbling quotes, highlighting, earmarking. I began consuming everything I could; I'd read a book, watch a film, then find the writer, actor, whoever online and reach out, which would lead me to another article, something else to watch.

I was realising as well that there were actually *words* for all my hunches, suspicions and feelings, a new vocabulary. Everything I was going through that I hadn't had the words for. Learning this changed me, radicalised me. It allowed me to figure out where I stood in the world.

I felt connected to all these voices through reading their work, some that have now died. Reading and learning about generations of disabled people felt like a rite of passage. I found myself uncontrollably sobbing at some of what I read and watched. For the first time since being dropped into this new reality I felt seen, and I saw a part of me in every book I read.

I wanted to mark this shift, and I was in my mid-twenties, so – of course! – I went for a tattoo. I chose the word *crip* on the inside of my left ankle. A term co-opted from the derogatory *cripple*, and reclaimed with pride by disabled people, used to examine the oppression of disabled people in society, throughout history. I wanted to be stamped with this understanding, our history.

My friend carried me while the tattoo artist, who got more than he bargained for, hauled my wheelchair up three flights of stairs.

My friend and I giggled uncontrollably; it was our first tattoo. I held my leg down, as the tattoo artist pressed the gun into my skin. It was the first time in a long while I had done something to my body that was my choice. And God, it felt good.

I realised there were pockets of community everywhere. I only have to look around a disabled seating area at an event, a place I was originally so uncomfortable with, and see faces I recognise.

I had a breakthrough when I went to my first festival as a wheelchair user. I had trepidations, visions of being stuck on the wheelchair platform, away from the crowds, unable to dance like everyone else.

I had woken up with the same old nerve pain, and I almost didn't go, worried it would bring up raw grief of things that I had lost. But I forced myself out of the house.

I could look at the people running and dancing and feel grief, but there was no yearning, rather a nostalgia for that time in my life that I ran and climbed. I could remember the person I had been, but that wasn't me any more.

I was unsure whether to go on the accessible platforms, but I found the grass limited my movement and couldn't see over anyone's waist, let alone get a glimpse of the stage. I swallowed my pride.

I was worried about people looking at me, as if they wouldn't be more interested in watching the headliner. But I felt an instant relief rolling up the ramp to the raised platform, finally able to see properly.

There was a man going around fist-bumping everyone. I saw a guy with cerebral palsy that I'd met earlier, and we waved to each other. The ground was smooth, making it easy to weave in and out. There was a woman in a glittery cape, driving her power wheelchair in and out of the lines of chairs, accelerating to the front of the platform when the music reached its climax.

I have come home to this place. What a difference a community makes, or, I should say, a willingness to open up to a community. Finding this collective felt like finding power.

Until so recently, disabled people were almost entirely excluded from society. In so many cases we still are. Talking about access to a gig suddenly feels inconsequential, pales in comparison to what people like me, who lived not that long ago, have suffered. Segregated, institutionalised.

How hard disability activists like Harriet McBryde Johnson and Judith Heumann, in the sixties and seventies, had to fight, just to have access to the same education.

Where would I have been if I had been injured in a different era? Certainly not a doctor.

A few times I have been in conversations with friends when they have imagined for fun their roles a hundred years ago, or throughout the ages, fantasising wild scenarios of kings, queens, sorcerers. When they turn to me, I feel like I dampen the mood when my response is that I would be dead or in some kind of institution. I can't help myself! That is the likely reality.

How many stories have gone untold? How many people have lived and died unseen? I think about all the people we've lost, through the years. Pushed to the outskirts, silenced, excluded from social events, not represented in anything we watch. Our voices erased from the narrative.

What privilege, what joy now then to be able to connect with others around the world, especially through the online communities we've formed.

I am so appreciative of everyone who has fought these battles, and to those allies and campaigners who continue to fight.

Independence is a fallacy

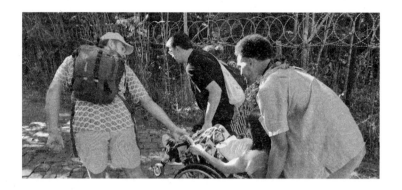

As a child, I loved to be described as *fiercely independent.* I wanted to do everything on my own; it would be proof I was capable, valuable. I wanted to be independent above all.

My definition of the word has changed dramatically, in the years since my injury.

During my inpatient stay at Stanmore, our newly introduced wheelchairs were moved from our bedside to the corridor every night until morning, to leave more room for nursing staff to come and go.

It took me years to recognise the irony of this. How would we ever be able to see the wheelchair as a tool for our independence, if it was made clear how easily it could be taken away from us? How easily we could be left stranded?

It was a message early on in my life as a disabled person that my autonomy is not a given any more, that it often comes with caveats. I now know that my basic needs can be stripped away at any moment.

I've heard that the hospital has stopped this practice since I left, thankfully, but the psychological impact was immense. It made me acutely aware that I am more vulnerable to infringements on my personal space, on my freedom.

I was learning that the grasp I had on my external environment was unstable.

One cold dark afternoon, I had a wheelchair skills session with my occupational therapist, Fran. I was trying to push around the outside of the gym building. We were working on flipping up my front wheels on to kerbs, weaving up and down slopes, manoeuvring across rough surfaces. She was explaining how I would have to plan my route as I wheel. Considering the state of London streets, the shattered pavements and potholes, I wondered how I would ever manage to do this on my own. Everything felt so impossibly hard, right then. While I was considering this, I felt myself going faster. Doubting my sudden increase in proficiency, I turned my head and saw that a stranger had appeared from behind, and she was pushing me.

Fran swivelled around, snapping at the stranger, telling her I was being taught to go up this ramp, that I needed to practise doing it on my own. This sharp tone was uncharacteristic for her and I was immediately aware that this wasn't an acceptable thing for this stranger to do. She protested that she was only trying to help.

This would not be the last time I would be pushed, pulled, picked up, carried without asking, all in the name of helping. Sometimes it's all too exhausting, and I let the tide of hands wash over me.

I have become painfully used to people who are *only* trying to help.

Rolling down the corridor in my first year as a doctor, another staff member that I didn't know came behind me and began to push me. It baffles me why she did this – she didn't even know where I was going! I felt totally passive, and so diminished.

People will jump at the idea of wanting to help me, assuming rather than asking what the best way might be to do this. Running for the door to hold it open no matter how many times I protest, that in fact it can be much easier for me to do it myself, rather than having to duck under an outstretched arm. I know that people just want to be helpful, but often it feels like they're doing this because they're uncomfortable seeing me doing things in my own way.

I wish people would just ask – and ask *me*, not the person I happen to be with.

I find that people often address whoever I'm with rather than asking me directly if I can walk or not, or what I might need. I am surprised how much this happens by default. Particularly when travelling – I am a body to be moved, not spoken to.

I have had to swat hands away as they dive in to grab my legs, lift me under my arms when I haven't even asked for any assistance. I sometimes wonder if it's because airport staff are so used to ferrying disabled people around, they no longer view us as autonomous humans, but as baggage to be handled.

To some people, my wheelchair signals that I am in a perpetual state of need. Of course, I have had to face the fact that I do need help at times. This was tough to reckon with at first. But requiring help doesn't mean I have to give up my right to be in control of what happens to my body.

I have learned, however, how much beauty there can be when we give up this attempt to do it all, to be independent, and accept the reality of our interconnections. While working on a respiratory ward on my second job as a doctor, I was inserting a cannula for a patient, D, who had motor neurone disease. He had no movement in his upper limbs. Thinking of my own legs, I gingerly touched and moved his hand and arm, looking for a vein.

We spoke about loss of mobility and the accompanying grief. He told me he used to enjoy fishing but could no longer do it.

My cannulation skills needed work and I was nervous. After some attempts I got the cannula in place and sighed with relief.

While I was cleaning D's hand and taping it up like a little present – my favourite part of the job – he asked me if I could see if a nurse was free. He'd been asking if someone could cut his nails for days, as they'd been digging into his hands. His fingers were folded in such a position that when his hands spasmed they pushed further into his skin, creating red crescent marks on his palms.

The nurse's desk had no nail scissors, so I took some normally used for cutting bandages back to his room and we attempted to tackle the nails. There was something special, to me at least, about us doing this together. Me, a doctor with no control over my legs trying to cut this man's nails, as he had no control of his arms. Together we'd just about make one able-bodied person. I could only do a rough job with the blunt scissors, but his relief was palpable.

'I can't feel them any more,' he said, smiling for the first time. 'Thank you, I really appreciate it.'

I could have cried. So often, as a very junior doctor, I felt like a tiny cog swallowed up in the huge machine that is the hospital. Completing hundreds of small tasks daily, while never having the sense that I was directly benefiting anyone.

This act felt valuable, as small as it was. I had been there myself, lying in bed desperately waiting for some basic need to be fulfilled, close to tears. In that moment they were my nails, my relief.

Some of the senior doctors in the mess joked that they wouldn't have done this. I smiled. They didn't understand what it feels like to have to rely on other people to live, to function. This was a special experience to be a part of: D had advocated for himself, and I was able to fulfil the task physically. He was the director and I was the actor. I wanted him to have complete control of what I was doing, how I was moving. I wanted it to play out exactly as he chose it to.

It's hard for some people to understand this particular dynamic. What do passers-by think when they watch my partner pushing me in my wheelchair along the street? I doubt that most see me as an equal member of the relationship. Even if I am telling him where to go, paying for the meal at the restaurant, supporting him emotionally. Do they see him as the hero for staying with me, and me as the burden? He is praised, I am grateful; he is resentful, I am indebted.

I have begun to realise that independence isn't my ultimate goal. I am looking for something else.

Alice Wong, a well-known disability activist, was one of the first people I heard define independence on the basis of *autonomy*, rather than physical ability. Alison Kafer in *Feminist, Queer, Crip* describes wanting 'interdependence not independence'. This is what I feel we should all be striving for.

I always appreciate an open offer from strangers directly asking me if I need help before they try. There's no need for apologising, no need to skirt around a question. 'You let me know if you need any help' gives me the power to decide, the control.

Any form of help that preserves my autonomy is the priority now. When someone reaches for something for me; sure that's helpful, but infinitely better if they can facilitate me being able to reach for it myself next time.

I am grateful to everyone who has done this and continues to do this. Enabling me to have choice, allowing me to lead the way by explaining what I need. Or to carry some of the burden; when I am running a teaching session with someone and a test fire alarm goes off and we realise there is no accessible route out, she emails afterwards to report it. She has experienced what a lack of access really means through my experience, and raised it as an issue, so I don't have to.

This is no passive state of dependence; there is a dynamism to my new life. My days now feel like an endless stream of mutual care. If they're able to, patients are eager to help me: pulling the blue curtain closed, pushing bulky NHS furniture out of the way, moving around in bed so I can reach them. They do things that I cannot do myself so that I can help them in turn. It is a constant to and fro of small acts we do together; we are partners in this. This is interdependence.

On a midnight shift, one of my front castor bearings explodes, so the next day Nathan and a close friend scour London in search of a skateboard repair shop to fix it. I'd had to finish my shift on three wheels, painfully aware I might topple over at any moment, if I leant too far to the left.

They do all this while I sleep, so I can be up for my next night shift and ready to get to work. They are the sole reason I am then able to make it to my shift and help a family whose father had just died, in confirming his death and talking to them about what happens next.

It is not just me sitting with them, but a stream of people behind me that have helped me get here, everyone that has come before.

Caring, but mostly being cared for, has changed me. It has forced me to become very good at advocating for myself. I have had to stop being a people pleaser, apologising for taking up space, and instead become patient, clear, firm, assertive.

Now I know how I will explain to a new work colleague how to pick me up and carry me up the steps of an inaccessible pub. Or instruct the black cab driver on how to use his newly fitted ramp. Or even on a night out, how to walk a friend through how to unpack and rebuild my wheelchair to put it in a taxi. I can make these things happen, knowing my boundaries, what I will and will not allow people to do.

I might have once believed this was admitting weakness, but I find strength in it now – my ability to advocate. There is something oddly reassuring to me to have experienced a loss of mobility. I am perhaps not as scared as others my age to get older, to become even more dependent. I am comfortable with being cared for in a way most of my friends couldn't imagine being. The past years have been lessons in accepting a reliance on others for my basic needs.

I can't pretend it's always easy. I know that I shouldn't feel like I'm a burden, but this is still something I must remind myself of again and again. That I am deserving of care. That my value in the world is not dependent on how much care I need.

There is an intimacy in all this too. I have become softer. I let strangers, acquaintances, friends hold me. I am close to people because I have to be. I have become more porous, more open. I have to tell people what I need. To be carried, pushed and pulled.

I remember when Nathan washed my hair for me while I was still in the Royal London, when I couldn't move my neck. It was greasy and knotted after nearly two weeks in bed. He covered my neck brace in towels to keep it dry, and then wet my hair with a bowl from the top of the bed. There's something lovely about someone washing your hair for you, as an adult. 'All I Want' by Joni Mitchell was playing in my head. His parents and mine were there, some friends too, laughing, talking.

These are moments of closeness that would never otherwise have happened – boundaries that have been broken down and rebuilt, differently. Would Nathan and I be as close if we had not had to go through this?

People around me work in synchrony, packing up my wheelchair into the car, lifting me into the sea, bumping me up steps. It is a dance we do every day with different variations. Lift, pull, reach. An endless flow of give and take – choreography that we know well by now. I turn on my front to sleep and Nathan, even if barely awake, instinctively feels my feet with his own to check they are not crossed, that they are not too cold.

I sit in a vast network of care.

I am always aware how much of a privilege it is that most of the care I receive is largely from my loved ones. I do not know how it feels to have a package of care provided by an agency, and I know from friends how difficult it can be to have it dictate your schedule, your life. To have strangers in your home, people you do not know, who you do not necessarily trust, helping with your personal care. Who come and go, and who may not do things correctly or fully understand your needs; who might arrive late, do not listen, do not make you feel safe.

But when it is done by someone you trust, whether

a professional or someone you're close to, there can be such a beauty in care.

There are moments when I am so grateful for my experience. How it has given me a deeper understanding of the nuance and intricate networks of care that sustain us all, the fluctuating nature of mobility and independence.

The pursuit of independence has been exposed to me as a fallacy. I don't want independence in the strict terms I always strove for as a child. If my life is made up of fleeting moments of connection and moments of kindness, I will be happy. I *want* to live dependent on others and I want others to depend on me. I cannot claim independence while seeking any type of comfort from others.

To be alive is to be dependent on one another; it is to be vulnerable, to be close to people, to know and fulfil each other's needs. If I am an island, I want all my loved ones on it with me.

These minute acts of care I experience daily are not only beautiful but radical. Care to me is the antithesis of capitalism. When someone lifts me into a car, helps me out of the shower, when I hold my friend's arm to help her balance, we are not here to make a profit or a product. We are here for each other. Caring goes against everything society seems to be hurtling towards. In a world that feels like it is becoming more and more hostile, to be kind is a profound act.

I have seen the best of people, time after time, as friends have showed up for me, given up their time and love to support me and help me out. When Juan turned up at my house, a few months after my discharge, he suggested we wheel to a café to chat, then took me to get a gym membership. I hadn't been coached by him for years at that point, and I hadn't been climbing for fun much at all, as I had been consumed by medical school. But my injury brought a new dynamic to our friendship, reinvigorated our bond. In what other circumstance would we have been able to have this relationship again? Where he could create exercise plans for me, motivate me? Where he could show love in so many new ways?

I have seen new sides to the people I love, in the past few years. About a year after my injury, I travelled to Australia to visit family. It was hard and navigating this new place as a wheelchair user. My aunt Sally is an occupational therapist; as soon as she heard that I was desperate to go in the ocean again, she found an old disused hospital wheelchair: I could transfer into it and then be wheeled into the ocean, slip out of it and swim. I loved her ingenuity, her creativity. It meant so much.

I could see her doing all she could to understand the way I moved now, and her experiences meant she really got it. We had long conversations about disability and mobility aids that would have been foreign to most people (and to me not long before). Suddenly we had a new, shared vocabulary.

In return, friends and family seem more willing to show their own vulnerability. Two years after my injury, I return to Istanbul as a wheelchair user when a close family friend, Hacer's husband, dies. It is her turn, now, to be vulnerable.

She is normally glowing, looking younger every time

I see her. Tonight, she is grey with grief. We walk down to Galata Bridge, past stray cats in shop doorways. We buy roasted chestnuts from a street seller and eat them on the way, cracking and peeling the burnt skin to reveal flesh that looks like a tiny brain and tastes like firm sweet potato. I gnaw on the blackened bits.

Hacer is laughing one minute and then sobs the next when she remembers.

We walk along the boardwalk of the Golden Horn to Karaköy, past mussel sellers. Whenever I reach a pavement drop or a step that my trusty electric wheel attachment can't handle, I find myself surrounded by Turkish men. They don't say anything, just come to help and then leave.

We meet with Hacer's stepson, Can (pronounced a little like John), who has Down's Syndrome, and is about fifteen years older than me. He has always taken on the role of a protector. I never thought we would be close. A nod hello was the limit of our interactions through my childhood. He doesn't speak English, and my Turkish is poor.

But on this trip, he wants to help carry me up the stairs, push me up the ramps, direct the traffic to let me pass. When we reach Hacer's, Can guides me into the lift in their apartment block. We get in and are both facing the mirrored wall. He stands behind me and puts his hands on my shoulders, leaning his face on top of my head and smiles. I rest my head on him and he holds it, kissing the top of my head. I want to cry at this gesture, this new understanding we have.

We are grieving the loss of his father together and finding new ways to communicate. I know he is someone who values hard work, and being helpful, and now I am a wheelchair user he has clear actions he can do for me: help push me up a ramp, divert traffic.

We have been given an opportunity of closeness we did not have before.

I have found this connection with strangers too – unique conversations with people I would not have had pre-injury.

I started volunteering at a food bank in lockdown because, like so many people, I was desperate to do something, and to feel like I had a place in a community. I found I could relate to some of the people who came in, who had somehow or other fallen out of mainstream society. We were alike in some ways; stigmatised to largely different degrees. This meant I was happy to tell them what had happened to me, if they asked. Because there were no platitudes involved, sometimes no surprise at all.

I remember once being on the reception desk, collecting information, when a man with a long, dark beard and a large coat came in, with no fixed address at the time, or NFA, as I tick on the form.

He sat down opposite me and told me immediately that he only wanted honey so he could have it in his tea. After reassuring him that we had honey, he relaxed a little and looked at me.

'So, you're in a wheelchair.'

The statement made me laugh. Yes, that's correct, I told him. He asked me why, and I gave him a two-sentence version of events.

'Life's weird, isn't it?'

I laughed again, very much in agreement.

While our circumstances are all different, and I'll never fully know the extent of the difficulties and judgement they face, like many of these people, I too have seen something of rock bottom. I have watched myself fall through a crack, lying below as others go on as normal. There is a shared understanding of rupture, of the earth under you breaking up to reveal something else. The realisation that you were never on steady ground to begin with. How fragile it all is, and how precious. There is solidarity in this.

My bodily state has an influence on people. Patients and strangers are honest with me now; people will tell me their deepest traumas when passing me in the street. I have learned to accept these admissions. Strangers who have been through things are drawn to others who have clearly been through something too.

I have found this understanding of grief, of difficulty, to be a gift at times. I feel I have been given something of a trading chip. People are open with me, sometimes almost instantly, like I have been given the password.

On an anaesthetics job as a first-year doctor, I would shadow an anaesthetist each day, helping with little jobs like flicking switches on the anaesthetic machine when asked, lowering and raising the bed depending on what the surgeon wants, marking the patient's oxygen levels and blood pressure and heart rate every five minutes neatly on a graph with an X, drawing up the milky white propofol to put someone to sleep.

I am in gynaecological theatre one afternoon shadowing a new anaesthetist, Tessa. We are listening to seventies rock (the consultant surgeon's choice) and the smell of burning flesh soon fills the air.

I like Tessa, she is calm and thoughtful. I notice she has a notebook with her, and every so often she jots something down. We start to talk about writing – writing for fun, writing for recovery.

She tells me her son had died by suicide a few years before, and how devastating that had been, and what she wants to write about now.

The surgery is laparoscopic, so they've inserted cameras into the patient's abdomen, and I can see on the two video screens the surgeon gleefully pulling apart a tightly coiled fibroid with a long, sharp metal grabber he has named *The Mother-in-Law*. 'It bites.' He grins at us.

While a somewhat gruesome scene is unfolding on the screens, we huddle around the glowing light of the anaesthetic machine, speaking in hushed tones about things that are deeply private.

People let me hold their grief, briefly, share their stories.

I have been forced to have honest, hard conversations with people close to me. Forced to feel uncomfortable, and through that discomfort, understood. Through that discomfort a new, stronger bond has formed.

Nathan, my family and I have had to navigate such unique situations because of my disability. I have had to be more honest than I have ever been, with how I feel, with what is important to me.

My life is undoubtedly more complicated, yes, but I

have seen sides to my family and friends I am not sure I ever would have otherwise. I have also had to recognise what matters, and what doesn't, and appreciate my life in a new light. Our relationships are so much deeper for that.

Arguing, shouting, crying, then laughing. It may be easier to ignore or avoid these tough conversations if you aren't forced to have them. But we have had them all. There is a greater depth to my interactions now. I do not want surface level any longer.

Early on I was so grateful to still be alive. I would whisper to myself, repeating *I am still in the room, I am still in the room.* I'd get goosebumps and feel a tingling at the back of my neck.

I live every day in the knowledge of my own mortality. I had not realised that being close to death can make you feel so much more alive. I better understand the fragility of life, the fragility of circumstance.

I write constantly, sending letters, notes. Pieces of permanence. For a long time, I acted around people like it might be the last time I saw them. I still try to not hold back.

Early on in hospital, I became fixated on the song 'Are You Ready for Love' by Elton John, and listened to it on repeat every night while lying in bed. I think I was so ready, so ready for love.

Since my injury I am so much more generous with my love, with my gratitude. I attempt to live a life without regret. I had to break in multiple places to understand this. I value relationships and friendships, over anything. Rich bonds, rich gratitude, rich grief.

I have had to be clear about what I need, not just with the people closest to me, but those I meet fleetingly. I have had to need people. This openness was not my choice, but it has led me to connections with strangers I would never have had otherwise. I connect to people so much more now; I can't hide my vulnerability.

The care dynamic opens up these opportunities for connection, for intimacy. Leaning my head on my friend's cheek as she gingerly carries me down the stairs. There is a time as a child where your parent will pick you up for the last time. But I have had to be carried by my mother and father again and again: upstairs, and into the car back when I couldn't transfer myself.

When else would I be held by my mother, and Sally, my cousin, in the sea to help me right myself after a big wave? I hold on to my father's foot in the rough current while he swims, dragging me back in to shore.

I am forced to be vulnerable, and it opens me up to these possibilities of connection. I have become a spider web of connections, a mesh of spindles that cocoons me. This injury has opened me up in ways I do not wish to ever close again.

Radical acceptance

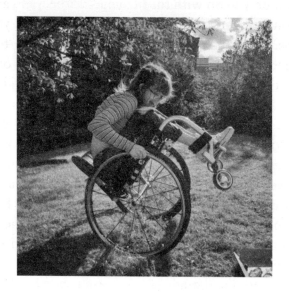

I spent so long not knowing who I would be after my spinal cord injury.

I desperately missed the boat we had been living on just before I went into hospital. Sure, I missed it because it was fun, but I think I missed it most because I equated it with youthfulness, spontaneity, naivety. This injury had come at a time when I was already changing, growing up, so maybe the hardest part was that I wasn't allowed to decide how quickly that would happen.

It was all incredibly painful at first – everything I tried to do, every experience I had, was through a lens of loss. Even the joy was painful. The passing of time felt so incremental at the start. Every day was exhausting, endless. I was grasping at straws of understanding, trying to make sense of the world and my place in it.

What do you do with the life you had planned, all the things that you've imagined for yourself, when everything changes? I had such vivid pictures of belaying my future children, teaching them to climb, spotting them on the wall. Scouring for cowrie shells on the Tasmanian beach by the old boat ramp, like I did with my mother.

But – walking along Regent's Canal looking at the people opening up their houseboats for the morning, thinking of my own time on our boat – I have come to realise you can yearn for things that you no longer want.

These imagined futures will be different now, but by no means worse. Rather, all of this has opened the door to feeling as though I can be even more than I envisioned for myself. The slate is clean now.

Sometimes the thought of my previous life catches my breath; I miss the ease of it all, the innocence of living in a body that does not betray me, that I cannot predict.

But then would I even appreciate it, if I still had it? Probably not.

Memories from before my injury seem like a different channel, a film screening of a different girl. They are barely imaginable to me now.

In my family, we still use my injury as a time stamp: pre and post to relate to the passing of time. It marks the end of an era, and the beginning of a new one.

I was determined to go back to places I used to love, to forge new memories in these spaces. Returning to somewhere untouched by my injury always causes me to go through the same cycle of grief again, although on a much smaller scale. It is a very, very peculiar feeling to roll where I once walked, but it is a seal that I need to break, until my body and the landscape match up again, find an equilibrium. It is important to me, to do this wherever I can, still.

I write this from a balcony in Turkey. Last time I was in this exact spot, pre-injury, Nathan and I were showing some friends the dance from *The Last Waltz* that Van Morrison does in his final song: you jump in the air and hit your feet together. I'd fallen over so hard, I thought I'd broken my hip. I laughed at the time, lying on the tiled floor. Youthful innocence.

It is different here now, because I am different.

Nathan piggybacked me across the rocks down by the sea. I would have told you it was one of my favourite places in the world before my injury; molten lava has created a scattered mosaic of bubbled rock surfaces so you have to jump from one to the other to reach the water. It was always a haphazard and risky route, and when I was little I once slipped down one of the gaps and ripped the skin from the entire side of my right leg. I can still see the scars in a certain light.

But today I had ridden my Batec handbike down to where the dusty road met the rocks and closed my eyes. Nathan carried me to the point where I used to jump in, but I felt nothing. Maybe this is a place from history now. All holiday I had thought how badly I wanted to find a way to get into the water there, but now, looking at it, I could see it was far too dangerous for Nathan to carry me any further down. There was a possible way to swim all the way round from a shallow rock pool, but it felt messy, undignified, unnecessary. I don't want to treat my body that way.

I used to dive down as deep as I could, but I could never touch the bottom. I used to collect sea urchins, large, spiky black spheres firmly attached to the rocks. You had to be very careful how you picked them off, gently holding on to the underside with your fingertips and twisting to release from the rock, I'd then go and create my own sea urchin community in a rock pool, watching them move about.

These places untouched by trauma, from the before time, seem innocent. Untarnished by pain but also by knowledge. I look back on the girl who last came here and see that she didn't know her place in the world, what she had a right to.

What happened here will now be replaced with new memories. New, more complex feelings than before. Grief will now find a place to settle here.

It feels like my own odyssey, the need to revisit these places, conquer them again from an entirely new point of view. Looking up at the people I used to be at eye level to. It is like a rite of passage for my new life, to fill up these spaces, to demand, to prove that I still exist here.

I have been forced to become someone I love. Learning to fix my wheelchair myself, learning to look after my body, finding things that make me feel the most alive.

New forms of fulfilment, of adventure, have arrived and filled up the space.

I believe a worn wheelchair is sign of a life well lived. The glue on the Velcro of my leg strap, which no longer works because I once wheeled into the swimming pool with it. Rust from being caught in the rain after a night out. Wheels whose grip has been rubbed down bare from skidding on concrete, dirt, sand, rocks, carpet, puddles, laminate flooring, wooden boards, grit, snow, autumn leaves.

Every time someone picks me up out of a car, bumps me up a step, helps me down a steep ramp, I am challenging a world that is not designed for me. But here I am, I want to shout. And I am not going anywhere. I am going to enjoy a life that society has told me is not worthy. That is activism.

Many people seem to believe that access that requires assistance from someone else is not true access. An example would be to use a ramp you must first call or press a button for someone to bring out a ramp. I do agree with this in some respects, but if I stuck to this principle, I know I wouldn't be able to go anywhere. I have learned I must be pliable to be allowed into these worlds, whether I like it or not.

I am also very lucky I am able to be this way: I can be lifted, I can clamber, drag, haul, transfer, fit myself into spaces that are not necessarily made for me. I cannot wait for the world to catch up with my ambitions, and maybe one day people like me won't need to work so hard, or struggle so much.

What is really special now is when I don't have to fight, to ask, to struggle. The feeling of true belonging, when it feels unconditional, undivided, consistent. Whether that's with other disabled friends, or friends that take on the responsibility to ensure access, or being in an environment that is completely accessible. Friends who, if I am not able to go somewhere, don't want to be there either.

Mia Mingus defines this very specific emotion as 'access intimacy', an 'elusive, hard to describe feeling when someone else "gets" your access needs. The kind of eerie comfort that your disabled self feels with someone on a purely access level . . . It could also be the way your body relaxes and opens up with someone when all your access needs are being met.'

With the right people, this is how I feel, and I know I can do anything.

I find a lot of adaptations that are made are somewhat short-sighted, short-term. Many changes were put in place for me on each placement as I was rotating through jobs as a doctor, but these immediately stopped when I left. Why can't we be more ambitious than this? Why can't we be aiming for a more complete, long-term shift? I remember being asked in detail how I would use a shower and toilet as they were going to make a new facility I worked in more accessible. I appreciated the concern, but surely I would not be the only disabled person using it? Was there no possibility that another disabled person would take my place?

Does increased accessibility not benefit us all? More exposure to different people, different voices? More people included in the conversation? If only we could all imagine more accessible futures.

To me, access is all about belonging. The times when I feel like I truly belong in this world are few and far between now, but that has made these rare moments even more valuable. To me it is a beautiful feeling to be fully included, when so often you are not. I no longer take this for granted.

Hampstead ladies pond has become one of those places for me. Sometimes it is the only place I feel like I can really breathe out. I feel so safe there, with Tanya the Lithuanian lifeguard, who has taken me under her wing. She used to be a professional synchronised swimmer and has been teaching me to be a stronger swimmer all year.

I enter the freezing water and suddenly all my body has to do is stay alive. It has become quite good at that now. I know this will be the bravest thing I have to do all week. Five minutes before I get in, my mind is wiped clean.

I am plunged into the cold waters by a plinth I transfer on to, which Tanya then lowers into the pond. Tanya watches me from the deck, commenting on my stroke, as I swim from one buoy to another.

'SCOOP! SCOOP GRACE! SCOOP! RELAX!'

She gestures with her arms wildly.

I practise treading water with my hands and then swim back to cling on to the buoy for a breather. When I want to get out, Tanya lifts up the rope sitting on the edge of the pond and I swim under, until I reach the plinth. I climb on and she spins the lever to raise me up. Once I'm out, she takes my hands and moves them in an arc.

'Like this,' she says as she scoops. 'Not like this!'

I leave feeling warm and glowing inside. The older women changing in the access area smile at me, include me in their conversations about cupping: 'they were doing it in the Mesopotamian era!' I feel a lot of affinity with these women, where perhaps my pre-injury self would have seen little to connect us.

I look around at the accessible changing area and there is a blind woman, a wheelchair user, someone using a walking stick, someone with long Covid, someone with chronic back pain.

When I swim a few months later I am amazed at myself. It no longer feels so cold. I swim to buoy two, then three, then back to one, then to two again. The tame ducks, used to their swimming neighbours, paddle by me. A moorhen perches on the buoy, in touching distance. Its gleaming black eyes watch me as I swim, head cocked.

I tip my head back, pushing my ears under the water. It is so calm that I feel like I can hear the undergrowth. I close my eyes and feel the deep, cool pond beneath me. I feel like part of it, part of nature.

I start swimming more and more, and it feels so much easier. I manage to swim all the way through winter for the first time. Plunging and floating in the icy water.

One of the other diligent lifeguards shouts out to me from the pontoon: 'Are you okay, Grace?' They all know me by name now, know what speed I like to be lowered into the water, how far I will swim. They cover my wheelchair with an umbrella when it's raining, put a towel over my cushion ready for me.

'Yes, yes I'm okay!' I shout back, grinning.

And I am.

Everything that at first was so hard, has become softer, easier. Opening my eyes to this new reality used to be so exhausting, to feel so bitter, like the cold that used to make my bones ache.

But now, it's true. I am more than okay.

I knew almost immediately that I wouldn't go back and change what happened to me. Early on it was a coping mechanism born from a simple reason: someone most likely would have died if I wasn't there to catch this man's fall head first. But it has become something entirely different over time. I wouldn't take a cure now if there was one. My identity now – the community I have, the friends I have made, the learning I have had to do, the rich complexity of my existence, the way my injury forces me into situations I would never have been involved with – that is all too valuable to reverse.

In her book *The Rejected Body: Feminist Philosophical Reflections on Disability*, Susan Wendell writes: 'I cannot wish that I had never contracted ME, because it has made me a different person, a person I am glad to be, would not want to have missed being, and could not imagine relinquishing, even if I were "cured".' I underlined the paper so many times when I read this, nearly breaking through to the next page.

I feel as though I have come home to my body. Why

would I want to leave home? I am anchored by this identity, by this reality, in a way I never felt before my injury. Self-assured. Tethered. On solid ground. Is that just a part of getting older? Or is it because I have been forced to build myself back from the ground up?

I look back on the young, vulnerable girl lying in hospital in the early days, and I ache for her. It is hard to think that there was a version of yourself that was so pliable, so lost. But more than this, I'm excited to meet all the different versions of me that are yet to come.

I returned to the ward where I'd spent those first five days after my injury, to meet a woman who was in a similar position as me, five years later. I was wondering what advice I could give. How could I even start to explain to someone what their life could look like? I remember how impressionable I had been, how much uncertainty had lain ahead.

We talked, and at one point she said she thought it would be better to cut off her legs and I laughed. I'd had the exact same thought in those early days. It is hard, to see someone at the very start of their journey, knowing there are many hard days to come. I try to tell her that her life will be good after this, that this grief will not always be so profound, so all encompassing.

She seemed reassured but I knew it was hard to believe. I did not always believe it at the time.

I just so strongly wanted to tell her this is not the end. That her life will still be what she makes of it. That she has no idea of the possibilities that lie ahead. That rehab will teach her how to function, but not how to live. I wanted her to know that she didn't have to accept a smaller life, or the constraints of the expectations and stereotypes she would face. I want her to know other people's opinions of her do not have to be hers to keep.

I felt so grateful that I could leave that place when we finished talking. That I didn't belong there now. I cycled back through Brick Lane and bought a box of doughnuts for myself on the way.

Every year I celebrate my *alive day*, the anniversary of my injury, the 17th of October. I co-opted the phrase from other disabled people who mark their own day to commemorate, to remember how far they have come. Some people I know treat it as a sombre day, a day for reflection, but I spend my life reflecting on every interaction I have, how it has changed now that I am disabled. What I want most is for the day to feel life-affirming, for me and everyone around me. I want to cherish them, to celebrate life.

How freeing it was to recognise this as a random event.

I cannot count how many people have told me that *everything happens for a reason* in response to my injury. I find it a pointless phrase, an inane response, though some might find comfort in it. I believe that nothing happens for a reason, but we make meaning from the random series of events that life throws at us.

What happened to me only confirmed this in my mind. To me, this isn't nihilistic, but hopeful. I have *made* meaning from this event. And this means I can make meaning from anything. Anything I choose.

It is not just an acceptance of the cards I was dealt,

and the unfolding events of the past five years, it is *embracing* them. It is jumping right in. It is actively joining a community, being part of something bigger than yourself.

It is a radical acceptance; hand in hand with a rejection of the deeply internalised and ignorant opinions many people still hold about disabled people. It is critically looking at how the infrastructure of our world perpetuates ableism, holds up ableist viewpoints, continues to devalue the existence of disabled and chronically ill people.

It is the conviction that it doesn't have to continue to be this way.

It is wholeheartedly believing the world, this society, could be better for us, and needs to be better for all of us. It is believing disabled people deserve MORE than this.

I know I will always be recovering. To me recovery is being open to growth and I always want to be open to growth, pliable to the ways my body has changed and will continue to change.

I will always hold grief and joy in two hands, but they have found a comfortable place to cohabit. What a privilege this has been so far, this journey. I never knew how far I would come. Is this the end? I think it's the start.

All I know is, really, I am richer for this.

Epilogue: On Fairness

Dear Miss Spence Green,

I am contacting you as you were a victim of a serious crime. The Victim Contact Service works with victims of serious and violent offences, where the offender is sentenced to at least 12 months in prison or given a Hospital Order.

We are contacting you to offer you the opportunity to have information about the offender in your case.

Please find attached a copy of our introductory letter, the Victim Contact Service leaflet & reply form.

If you have any questions or queries, please don't hesitate to contact us – I understand that this has been extremely difficult and I apologise if this email has caused you any additional anxiety or distress.

Kind regards,

Donna James
Case Administrator
Victim Contact Service – London NPS

It took me a long time to understand what exactly had occurred that day in Westfield. But it was already written the night of the 17th of October 2018, typed up and ready for the morning news.

MEDICAL STUDENT PARALYSED BY IMMIGRANT

After our collision in Westfield and a shared night in A&E, our paths did not cross again. My perpetrator, as he was described, became an unknown, shadowy figure in my mind. We would begin to refer to him ominously as 'The Man', and from then on, he would always be known by that name.

In those early days I worried that if I knew his actual name and used it, everything would become much more real than it felt. I wanted to know as little as possible, terrified every new bit of information I received would somehow incapacitate me.

Police officers came to film my account of the day a few days after my injury, to be played in court so I wouldn't have to be there.

The idea that I had any place in *court* seemed so strange to me. I couldn't quite understand how I had found myself in the middle of this, these large and serious processes occurring outside while I lay in this hospital bed.

My designated officer, Damien, asked me what I had done before I got to Westfield, and what I remember happening afterwards. He hesitated before asking his last question: had I seen the man who jumped before?

I was confused. I had still never seen him; he had collided with me from above. My first view of him would be in the newspaper many months later.

Damien said he had watched two hours of CCTV footage from Westfield. 'The Man' had smoked weed in the stairwell beforehand, and then taken a run up before diving over the third-floor balcony head first. I wanted to ask him what I looked like, lying on the floor. Were my legs twisted? Was I facing down? Was I still holding my bags? I couldn't picture myself there.

His injuries were minimal. He had been sectioned at a psychiatric hospital at first, but it had been determined that his intention wasn't suicide.

I didn't know how they could *determine* that, but as bizarre as the first event was, the dribs and drabs of random bits of information that followed were similarly baffling. None of it made any sense and that almost made it easier. It was as if it were a made-up story, a dream.

Journalists reached out to me for a comment. What did they expect me to say? I was supposed to have views on an event that I barely understood had occurred.

Through the haze of information, the realisation that I likely inadvertently saved his life by breaking his fall, helped me so much in those early days, when confusion was a heavy, thick cloud over my consciousness. The only thing I could hold on to, that I knew with absolute conviction, was that I wouldn't take it back. I wouldn't reverse the day. *If I wasn't there someone would have died*, I would tell myself over and over again. No matter who the man is or what he did, no matter that the choice made was not mine, I would make that same choice every time. A choice I would take hypothetically, is now something I live with.

Grace Spence Green

How could I be completely destroyed by something that I wouldn't reverse? I tried to reason with myself.

I was desperately trying to grab hold of a single morsel of understanding, of clarity. To find my footing in this new world I had landed in. 'Grace is a pragmatic individual who values certainty' wrote my inpatient psychiatrist in my notes.

Apart from this logic, what I actually felt was an absence of emotion. Was there something wrong with me? I worried it was all around the corner, all to come. I was waiting for a tsunami wave of bitterness and anger to wash over me, crashing through the numbness, because that was how I was *supposed* to feel, right? I could barely summon anything.

I felt only an overwhelming amount of assumed anger, and heavy was the burden of carrying everyone else's rage.

A nurse that worked at Stanmore when I was an inpatient there looked at me strangely one morning, like she wanted to tell me something that she shouldn't. She began to speak, and then hesitated, shaking her head. I pressed her, irritated by her indecision, my patience at an all-time low. Eventually she spoke.

'I would have killed him, you know.'

As if that must be what I am thinking too. As if that would help me in some way.

Taxi drivers have taken a more brash approach. 'I would have killed the *bastard*.'

I laugh at the naivety of this. How strangers are able to make it so simple! Even though it has not happened to them, some people are so sure of what they would do, how they would feel.

201

My story can bring out ugly reactions. Something unpleasant is dredged to the surface.

I used to worry that these ugly thoughts and emotions would catch up with me. That I was missing something everyone else could see. That I would one day be consumed not by grief or sadness, which I know well, but bitterness, jealousy, anger. I know now that I won't.

A year after the collision I finally saw the man's face, in an article a somewhat clueless friend had sent me. It looked like a mugshot: he has a blank expression, large brown eyes looking upwards at something not pictured. It is side by side with a photo of me smiling at a climbing competition years earlier, that I imagined some unpaid intern had had to trawl social media to get hold of.

I only caught a glimpse before I quickly swiped away, shaking. For the past year I had thought that if we were face to face, it would tear my entire world down. I thought the weak scaffolding that I had built up around my consciousness over the months would disintegrate. But I felt nothing. I was not afraid, and I realised I never had been.

I told Juan what had happened, and he texted back: that's FUCKING AWESOME! He said he didn't know how he'd feel if he saw the face of the man that attacked him thirty years ago in Venezuela. But perhaps that's different.

I wasn't attacked, I wasn't targeted. I was in a place at a time, and something occurred. The age-old *wrong place wrong time* can't apply as I wouldn't change my place or time within it.

By now, I have seen his face more times than I can count. People find it hard to understand that I think of him so little, that for him to cross my mind someone else must mention him. There is an assumption we are somehow inextricably linked now and for ever, that I must have a relationship with him. That I must know him intimately.

I seem to be the only one not interested in the answer of *what was he trying to do?* No matter his motivations, they do not change my feelings. I feel certain in this. Whether he thought he could fly, or the psychiatrists were wrong and there were suicidal intentions, it does not alter my reality. No matter his intentions – it does not change the resulting chain of events. His is not my story to tell. It does not alter where I have ended up in this, or where I will go.

My victim support officer Donna, a friendly lady, came to meet me twelve months down the line to explain the next steps, asking if I wanted to meet him. She said it could be helpful if there were any questions I wanted answered, but I didn't. Strangers I have told seem to ruminate on it more in one brief conversation than I have done in years. I'm not interested in any kind of television moment – a moment of restorative justice. The perpetrator faced with the victim, the questions answered, case closed. A classic story of someone wronged, someone else punished. Neat vindication.

My God, is it more complex than that.

I started speaking publicly about how I felt and about this complexity, only to find in the headlines the next day: MEDICAL STUDENT FORGIVES MAN FOR JUMPING ON HER.

How do I argue that there is no forgiveness because there was no anger in the first place? The next thing I tend to hear is:

That is so unfair
Was it unfair?

I swerve away from that word, wanting to let it brush off my body. How completely unjust that a young white girl who was at medical school was crushed by a black immigrant man who was smoking weed. On some level, I think that's what people are really saying.

To call it unfair suggests it should have happened to someone else. Should he have died instead?

It opens the door to the cesspool of 'what ifs'. What if I was two seconds earlier and watched him hit the floor head first in front of me? What if he landed on a different person? What if he never jumped in the first place? But he did. None of these scenarios exist: they disappear before my eyes. They are smokescreens.

If I am humouring these imaginary potentials, I must also consider the real possibility I could have died that day. I cannot consider one without the other. That put to bed the agonising ruminations quite quickly as I lay in hospital. I stopped picking at that scab.

What even is fairness? Is it fair that because of the economic circumstances and the social class I was born into, I can afford the financial hit of disability, unlike so many others? That I don't have to rely on benefits, that I can afford therapy, that I can afford physiotherapy, that I can afford the frankly outrageous price of a good wheelchair?

Socio-economic factors are more disabling in so many ways. Class underpins everything. With class comes social capital, connections, friends or contacts to give knowledge, support. Money.

My experience of disability is starkly different from someone who does not have this safety net. Having to rely solely on a social system that has been degraded by austerity and underfunding is a prospect I do not have to face.

So when people say, as they often do, *That guy just got to walk off and ruined your life*, what happened might have actually ruined his. He was was sentenced to four years, released after serving two, and then deported. I asked if there was anything I could do to stop his deportation. I didn't want this event to cause any more damage, any more harmful ripples, but it was out of my control.

His act nudged me in a new direction, but I am still doing the career I love and have learned to take advantage of the sensational nature of my injury as a platform to talk about issues I care about deeply. As different as our paths were prior to the collision, they remain very different now.

There has been horror and grief that has buckled me at times, but so many things have been in my favour, allowing me to succeed. The cards have not been stacked against me. My network has buoyed me.

I was made acutely aware of this recently. I was on my last shift as an F2 doctor, seeing newly admitted patients in A&E. I was rushing around the acute admission unit, a sort of waiting bay patients go to before moving up to a ward. On a bad day I would call it a purgatory.

A young man, C, who looked a similar age to me, was lying in one of the beds, watching me as I passed back and forth around the ward. At one point we made eye contact and he almost shouted: Please! Please can I talk to you?

I sighed inwardly, seeing patients that are not yours is never good. I knew I wouldn't be able to do much for him, but he seemed desperate. I wheeled over and instead of a request I was surprised to hear him tell me that he'd had a spinal cord injury three years ago. I was surprised, by the way he talked: he appeared to me a newly injured person. I was reminded of myself in the Royal London. We had similar levels of injury, but he could not believe the things that I could do on my own. He had carers coming in three times a day, and he was only able to do minimal things independently. He had never been to a rehab hospital; he had lost his place when he was going through some other challenges.

I tried to give C some advice before I left, I gave him details to Back Up, but I felt useless. He wasn't my patient, and it was my last day working at that hospital.

I was humbled. As hard as Stanmore had been, I was grateful to have learned so much there. It forced me into a rehab process that I was realising perhaps was always going to be hard, always painful, but worth it for the knowledge I had come out with, the foundation I was given to grow from.

I sat two metres away from C as he lay in bed but the gulf between us was far greater. The chasm appeared insurmountable to him, as impossible as learning to walk again. I had had an army behind me. My mother, intent on making sure I got to all my scans on time, which were always in some obscure corner of the hospital, acting like my own personal porter. My father, methodically sorting out all my life admin as everything went on hold, making notes in every meeting I had with various professionals. Nathan, an unflinching constant.

I realised that at every obstacle through my recovery I had been bolstered, whereas he had sunk deeper.

It sometimes feels as though to succeed as a disabled person you must have everything else lined up in your favour. Add in any marginalising factors or challenges, and things become exponentially harder – race, gender identity, sexual orientation, or poverty, lack of family or partner, lack of secure housing, uncertain immigration status, alcohol or drug dependency, mental health problems . . .

Sure, some of my determination and character have helped, and I have worked hard, but I also have a vast amount of privilege that has enabled me to have this life. I am part of a system which has enabled me to succeed, and which sets up so many others to fail. Mine is hardly a story of individual tragedy, or individual success or triumph. It's what happens when a community is found, when a person is loved, supported and given the freedom to learn, to hope, to change.

Resources

Back Up

Back Up is a national charity that inspires people affected by spinal cord injury to get the most out of life.

Back Up's services are designed by and are for people affected by spinal cord injury. Back Up teaches practical skills and gives confidence to positively adjust to life following spinal cord injury:

- Speak with others in a similar situation
- Multi-activity courses for daily life skills
- Family support
- Online courses
- Returning home from hospital
- Support returning to education, volunteering or employment
- Wheelchair skills training

Get in touch:
020 8875 1805
www.backuptrust.org.uk

Books

Disability Visibility by Alice Wong

Too Late To Die Young by Harriet McBryde Johnson

Sitting Pretty by Rebekah Taussig

Feminist Queer Crip by Alison Kafer

Being Heumann by Judy Heumann

Nothing About Us Without Us by James Charlton

Acknowledgements

There are people that helped me write, and there are people that helped me recover. Many overlap. Writing and recovering; neither were a solo project.

Nathan, it is impossible to measure the support that you give me; you do small things every day that make my life inconceivably easier and better.

You jumped into the unknown with me, and I am so grateful for the life we have built. I don't think you need to read this book, you've lived it.

Thank you to my parents for their unflinching support and love. None of this – and I really mean none of this – is possible without you two. It was my wonderful upbringing that equipped me with the skills to enable me to recover from this injury.

Thank you to Noemi for being a source of guidance and hope – I will treasure those conversations. To Juan for your honesty, commitment and friendship. For pulling me out of my rut. Thank you to Hatty for being there on the day, and every day since. To all my friends, I hope you know who you are. Everyone who sat in that hospital canteen, who carried me, lent me books, argued for me, laughed, cried with me.

Thank you to Dr Sam Thenabadu, Dr Tim Lancaster,

Dr Despo Papachristodolou and Dr Richard Phillips for making my return to medical school possible. Thank you to Mr Ivan Tomasi, Ms Sarah Wheatstone, Dr Alice Roueche and Dr Amelia Hughes for all the support and tools necessary to survive the first year of work as a doctor. To Lizzie Ferris for that phone call that made me realise it was possible.

Thank you to Vince and Rubes for being the best ward neighbours I could have asked for, and to the team at Spinal Crap for those early special conversations.

Thank you to Joanna and Clare for being my silent supporters, enabling me to get all the equipment I needed when I was discharged, so I could focus on the important things.

And for the ones lost while writing this book, Joanna and Yucel. Thank you both for giving me a beautifully different way to see the world.

To everyone who supported my family during this time, I am eternally grateful. I have been buoyed by a group of people, thank you to everyone on my islands.

Thank you to Fran, my editor, for believing in me, for imagining this before even I could. For your guidance and patience over the years. I couldn't have asked for a better person to do this with. Thank you to Ana Fletcher for your vital early input.

And to the rest of the wonderful team at Wellcome and Profile Books, I feel so proud to be a part of your work.

Thank you to Jacquie Drewe and Gordon Wise at Curtis Brown for always advocating for me.

To Rebekah Taussig, Judy Heumann, Mia Mingus,

Alice Wong, Alison Kafer, Eli Clare, Harriet McBryde Johnson, Tom Shakespeare, Mike Oliver and Nina Tame for your words and stories. They offered the hands to grab a hold of at a time when I felt so lost.

Thank you to Mara for keeping me my body strong during this time. To the staff at my local cafe, particularly Helen, for keeping me watered and fed and humouring me spending six hours at the same table with one coffee. To Habibi, Biber and Minnoş for being the best lap cats a writer could have. Thank you to the Pademelon, a furry little marsupial who sat by my window watching me, for the last month that I wrote this in Tasmania.

And thank you, most of all, to the disabled community.